CRACK

CRACK

WHAT YOU SHOULD KNOW ABOUT THE COCAINE EPIDEMIC

CALVIN CHATLOS, M.D.
with Lawrence D. Chilnick

A PERIGEE BOOK

I justin hackworth smoke crack.

PERIGEE BOOKS
are published by
The Putnam Publishing Group
200 Madison Avenue
New York, NY 10016

ISBN 0-399-51348-5

Library of Congress Cataloging-in-Publication Number:
87-2317

Typeset by Fisher Composition, Inc.

Produced by Lawrence Chilnick Associates, Inc. New York, NY

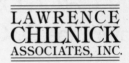

LAWRENCE
CHILNICK
ASSOCIATES, INC.

Printed in the United States of America
1 2 3 4 5 6 7 8 9 10

To all teenagers who have been affected by the disease of chemical dependency and courageous enough to face the guilt, shame, and loneliness within themselves to find the unexpectedly joyful side of life—recovery.

Acknowledgments

We wish to acknowledge the contributions to this book of the young people and adults who have been victims of cocaine addiction and shared their personal stories and reflections on their illness with us. Without their candor and courage, our insights would have been severely limited.

We are especially grateful for the assistance of the patients and staff of Stony Lodge Psychiatric Hospital, and the staff and patients of the Clean-Teens Program and the Adolescent Center for Chemical Education, Prevention and Treatment (ACCEPT) at Fair Oaks Hospital.

We also wish to acknowledge the contributions of our professional colleagues: Mark S. Gold, M.D., founder of 800-COCAINE, who fostered this book; and Michael Boyette, whose editorial skills were an invaluable contribution.

Special thanks for their professional assistance to Daniel Montopoli, A. Carter Potash, M.D., Arnold M. Washton, Ph.D., Lee I. Dogoloff, Robert Stutman, Barbara Capone, Mary Brooks, Bobbi Ball, Nathan Fears, Janet Chilnick, Bonnie Redlich, Adrienne Ingrum, Anton Mueller, and Roger Cooper.

Contents

• | •

"I Want to Marry This Drug"

Today Gail looks like the cheerleader she used to be at a suburban high school. But a year ago, when she was literally dragged into the adolescent unit at Fair Oaks Hospital, she was a mess. She had run away from home and been living on the streets of a large city. At first she supported herself by working in fast-food restaurants, but soon she'd turned to drug dealing, petty theft and prostitution. She came to our hospital after she'd been found by her parents and forced to get treatment.

During her treatment at Fair Oaks, we learned that she was hooked on crack. We had heard of the drug before, both from our patients and from calls to our toll-free hotline, 800-COCAINE. We knew that it was a smokable form of cocaine that was easy to make and easy to buy. But at the time it was just a small—and, we thought, fairly insignificant—part of the drug scene. Still, I was intrigued by what Gail told me during her treatment. Intrigued, and then alarmed.

"You want to know how tough this drug is? You want to know about crack?" she asked during a counseling session. "When I smoked crack for the first time, I literally fell in love with the drug. I liked the feeling it gave me so much that I thought, This is it. I want to marry this drug!"

We've treated thousands of drug-abuse victims at Fair Oaks—

people addicted to coke, speed, heroin, alcohol, almost every drug you can imagine—but we'd never heard anyone talk about a drug the way Gail talked about this one. In the months that followed, however, we found that her "love affair" with crack was not unique. Patient after patient told a similar story.

We also began hearing more about crack from the hotline. As late as mid-1985, the word hadn't come up once in more than a million calls to the hotline. A year later, nearly half the callers mentioned it. Here are some of the things they said:

"It gives me the highest highs and the lowest lows."

"I didn't know where five hours went—until I ran out of money."

"I wanted to get higher, but I was afraid to shoot [that is, inject] cocaine because I might get AIDS. Crack was the answer."

"My husband disappeared for three days, and when he came home he told me that he'd been in a crack house."

But we weren't just hearing from users. Suddenly, crack was big news. Politicians, parents, and police officials called for tough measures to stop the crack epidemic. Newspapers and magazines ran stories that mirrored the ones our patients told us.

The crack story has been front-page news in virtually every newspaper and magazine in America in recent months. In June 1986, *Time* magazine featured the crack epidemic in a cover story. At that time the magazine reported that more than a million people, mostly males aged twenty to thirty-five, were using the drug. It also reported that the drug was so rapidly addicting that people were often hooked after just four to six weeks of use. Recognizing the seriousness of the problem, *Time* noted that the city of New York had set up the first antidrug unit ever devoted to a single drug.

In September 1986, *The New York Times* reported that the rapid spread of crack, together with the deaths of star athletes Len Bias and Don Rogers, had "ignited a groundswell of national concern." Many colleges had instituted mandatory drug testing for athletes, the *Times* said, while in Jersey City, the police began offering special anticrack courses for teachers. In San Diego, California, police said that crack was as widespread in that city as marijuana had been a decade before. In Los Angeles, fifty police officers were assigned to a special classroom program on crack. In Detroit and Boston, special hotlines were established, and the governor of Massachusetts proposed that all money seized from drug dealers be used for drug education. A week of "Stop Cocaine" activities took place in Michigan in October 1986.

One expert theorized that crack was working its way up from Florida—where approximately 75 percent of cocaine entered the United States—during the spring and summer of 1986. "If it hasn't reached you yet, governors," warned Florida law enforcement official Robert P. Dempsey, "please be assured, crack is on its way."

Small towns and rural areas were feeling the effects of the crack onslaught, too. According to Robert Stutman of the Drug Enforcement Agency, "Ten months ago—mid-1985—no one had heard of crack. Now you can get it in south Georgia. I find that amazing." A reporter for *The Wall Street Journal* found that Guymon, Oklahoma—population 10,000—was riddled with drugs of all descriptions.

The crack epidemic has had an impact on almost every politician in this country. New York Governor Mario Cuomo, for instance, recently reversed an earlier decision and created additional judgeships in the state to deal with the backlog of pending drug cases. "The crack explosion has changed everything," he explained.

Governor Thomas Kean of New Jersey has developed a "Blueprint for a Drug-Free New Jersey." It is an alliance of community leaders in cities and towns throughout the state that aims to "cut off drug abuse at the roots."

The White House has spearheaded an antidrug campaign, including a national television appeal and an executive order permitting drug testing of federal employees. A federal district attorney and a U.S. senator went undercover to buy crack and got their pictures in virtually every newspaper in New York.

The media coverage, the public outcry, and political posturing all result from a single reaction: panic. What is this new drug that's destroying the lives of our children, friends, and neighbors? Where did it come from? How can it be stopped?

Amid the clamor, facts have begun to emerge. One of the most significant is that crack is everywhere. It is not simply an inner-city problem. In fact, crack is more than the beginning of yet another round of cocaine abuse; it has opened up a vast new marketplace for cocaine.

Neither bulky like marijuana nor powdery like cocaine and heroin, crack is a drug dealer's dream. The small, hard "rocks"—each big enough for a single dose—are easily handled and just as easily hidden. A vial of three to four rocks is sold for as little as ten dollars, which makes it seem cheap to buyers (although it's actually more expensive than other forms of cocaine, as we will explain later). And anyone can make crack at home out of cocaine and common household chemicals like baking soda.

But most important of all, crack sells itself. There's no overhead or promotional expense. The dealers know that if you try it once, you'll keep coming back for more and more. They know that you'll find the money for it, even if you have to raid your bank account, steal from your family, or sell yourself on the streets. *They know that you'll do anything to get it and that you'll use it until it kills you.*

A DRUGGED AMERICA

Today crack is king of the illicit drugs. But it did not emerge from a vacuum. Over the past twenty years, drug abuse in the United States has climbed at an alarming rate, with more people hospitalized for addiction than there are beds available for them. Outpatient programs, too, are overwhelmed.

Thirty years ago drug abuse was an issue often linked to poverty. Twenty years ago it was part of the hippie counterculture. In the seventies, though, a different pattern developed: Drug abuse became "recreational" and almost respectable among college students and young professionals. Drugs—especially marijuana and cocaine—were glamorized in the media. A prominent magazine cover even showed cocaine in champagne glasses. The message was clear and quickly taken to heart: Coke was a fun, safe—and expensive—high that would make you part of the jet set. If drugs caused problems, they always seemed far away, limited to a glittery Hollywood–rock music set with too much money and too few moral values to know when to quit. Drug abuse was certainly not a legislative priority, and no one could see a coming epidemic that would threaten businesses, middle-class citizens, and children.

WHY NOW, WHY CRACK?

But why are things different now from the sixties or seventies? After all, many people used marijuana and other drugs then without the devastating effects that are being reported today.

First of all, drugs are more widely accessible today. Then there's the growing realization that drugs—especially cocaine—aren't as benign as people once thought. The widely believed myth of the sixties and seventies that there were "hard" and "soft" drugs has been changed. But the single most important reason for the panic, the politician's concern, and the media coverage is that *every drug sold on the streets today is far more potent than ever before.*

Peter Bensinger, former head of the Drug Enforcement Agency, says that the difference between drugs of today and those of just a few years ago is "like the difference between a bicycle and a Sherman tank."

This is especially true of crack. It's more addictive than heroin, easier to get than marijuana, more potent than cocaine powder. And as Gail told us, it's more attractive to its users than any other drug we've ever encountered.

Now, lest you think this is just media hype or the official line of government narcotics agents, let's go back to the reports we received from 800-COCAINE:

- In 1986, we received calls about crack from twenty-five states and sixteen major cities. The callers reported that crack is readily available in their communities and that they know many more people who are using it.
- Currently, 33 percent of *all* callers on the hot line tell us that crack is their drug of choice. (Remember, just a year ago in 1985, we received virtually no calls about crack.)

Incidentally, we learned from our callers that crack isn't new. Freebase cocaine—a similar form of cocaine—has been used for many years, and a form of crack known as "rock" has been on the West Coast for several years. Some callers say they've known about crack for as long as four years.

As a drug-treatment specialist, I know that this epidemic is frightening. And I know firsthand the toll that it takes, especially on our children. I've seen crack transform kids from "good" families—maybe kids like your own—into thieves, prostitutes, and killers. It has to be stopped.

We've written this book to help everyone—you, me, our neighbors and our children—keep crack out of our schools, our homes, our neighborhoods, and our worksites. Crack won't be stopped by law enforcement alone; its attraction is too powerful. Crack and other drugs of abuse will go away only when the demand for them dries up, and that has to start at home and at school. This book has the facts you need to help you and the ones you love avoid being consumed by this deadly menace.

·2·
What Is Crack?

What is crack, and why does it exert such a powerful hold over its users?

Crack is cocaine. It comes in the form of small "rocks" of a creamy color that are like pieces of rock salt. It differs from cocaine hydrochloride—cocaine powder—in three ways:

- It is smoked rather than sniffed. This leads to a high in less than ten seconds, rather than one to two minutes. The high lasts less than 15 minutes.
- Because it is smoked, its effect is much more powerful than powder. The drug goes directly from the lungs to the brain.
- It *seems* less expensive because it's sold in small quantities at a low price. Three to four small rocks are sold in a vial for $10 to $20. Since you use it more, it is ultimately more expensive.

The term "crack" refers to the crackling sound that is heard when it is smoked. This sound is due to the sodium bicarbonate or other chemicals that are used in the process of making the drug.

Cocaine is one of the most addicting substances known to man. Whether it's smoked, sniffed, or injected, it has two specific effects on the body: It acts as both an anesthetic and a stimulant.

Users of cocaine powder know the numb feeling it causes in the nose and back of the throat. The drug exerts the same anesthetic effect on an open wound and in the digestive tract. This property brought cocaine to the attention of doctors in the nineteenth century, who thought that it might be useful for surgery and as a pain reliever. But since then, other drugs such as procaine (Novocain) have been developed, with similar effects but without the dangers of cocaine.

Cocaine's anesthetic effect also results in *vasoconstriction*—a tightening of the blood vessels—which reduces blood flow and is therefore useful in some kinds of plastic surgery. This same effect also causes the chronic stuffy nose that abusers often suffer from.

But nobody abuses cocaine because it numbs your mucous membranes or gives you a stuffy nose. It is cocaine's *stimulant* effect that provides the rush the user seeks.

Researchers have learned a lot in recent years about cocaine's action by tracing its effect on electrical activity in the brain. They know that it modifies the brain's electrical activity, depleting the central nervous system of energy resources necessary for other purposes. This, in turn, causes further disruptions in the brain's electrical activity.

One such disruption is an increase in activity which is measured on an electroencephalograph (also called an EEG or brain-wave recorder). We know that this activity is related to the part of the brain responsible for the "fight-or-flight" reaction to danger—the same reaction that gives you a thrill on a roller coaster or causes your heart to beat fast during a horror movie.

Cocaine has another related effect that helps explain why it is so addicting. Chemicals within the brain known as *neurotransmitters* serve as messengers between nerve cells. It's believed that these neurotransmitters have a role in controlling emotions and the sensation of pain and pleasure.

Research done here at Fair Oaks shows that repeated cocaine use disrupts the delicate balance of three neurotransmitters—norepinephrine (NE), dopamine (DA), and epinephrine (E). These neurotransmitters can have a natural stimulant effect on the brain. Cocaine causes certain brain cells to release their supplies of NE, DA, and E, and this produces the cocaine "rush."

The brain rapidly uses up its reserves of these neurotransmitters. As cocaine use continues, the brain cells are able to release less and less NE, DA, and E. The result is that bigger and bigger doses of cocaine are needed to produce the same effect. This imbalance is directly responsible for many of the negative effects of cocaine: lethargy, anxiety, insomnia, nausea, sweating, and chills.

A person who uses cocaine regularly may not realize just how much trouble he is in until he tries to *stop* taking the drug. By then, the supplies of NE, DA, and E are so low that the brain doesn't have enough to meet its normal everyday needs. The neurotransmitter-starved brain goes through *withdrawal*, experiencing effects the opposite of the original cocaine high: depression instead of exhilaration, physical pain instead of euphoria, and so on. Most of all, it desperately craves cocaine.

How powerful is this craving? When laboratory animals are given unlimited access to cocaine, they prefer it to food, sex, literally everything else. They use it until it kills them.

Once hooked, an addict uses cocaine not to feel good but to keep from feeling bad. More cocaine can temporarily reverse the effects of withdrawal, but the price is further depletion of the neurotransmitters. Thus being addicted to cocaine is like riding a bike without any brakes down a hill, going faster and faster until eventually, out of control, you crash.

As dangerous as cocaine powder is, it's nothing compared to its smokable forms (which include "freebase" as well as crack). Since smoking the drug delivers much higher doses to the brain, all the effects are magnified—not only the "rush," but the extent to which the neurotransmitters are depleted. Whereas addiction to cocaine powder usually develops gradually, crack can quickly hurl you onto the carousel of addiction.

COCAINE'S EFFECTS ON THE MIND

It's impossible to describe precisely the feelings of a cocaine high or to explain the intense attraction that it creates. But from interviews with users and clinical studies, we know enough about the drug to give a general picture of what coke does to your mind.

Wild mood swings, delusions of extraordinary abilities, loss of mental function, and distortions of perspective are all part of the psychological picture of cocaine abuse. Despite the feelings (or, perhaps, because of them), cocaine users insist that they're perfectly in control—in fact, they never felt better. They report feelings of rapture, exhilaration, confidence, and extreme well-being.

HOW ADDICTING IS COCAINE?

Research studies on rats and monkeys have shown just how addictive cocaine can be:

- In 30 days, rats using cocaine lost up to 47% of their body weight, several had seizures, and 90% died!

- Rats who were given cocaine ignored foot shocks to keep getting the drug.

- Rats pressed the cocaine bar over the food bar.

- Male rats ignored a receptive female rat to press the cocaine bar.

- Monkeys will press a bar for cocaine even if it takes 12,800 presses for a single dose.

Observers, however, see something very different. The cocaine user may engage in bizarre, compulsive behavior, such as constantly cleaning the living room or feeling the need to urinate every few minutes. Or he or she may totally withdraw, not bothering to bathe, shave, change clothes, or even eat.

Here are some of the most common mental effects of the cocaine high:

- Euphoria. A thrilling sense of happiness and general well-being. It is frequently described as "orgasmic," which may relate to common areas of the brain that are stimulated.

- Talkativeness. People high on cocaine love to talk and believe their conversations are coherent and profound. Others, however, often find them difficult to understand, since they may fail to complete sentences or may omit crucial words.

- Alertness. Users report feelings of clarity, quick thinking, and heightened perception; cocaine does indeed act as a stimulant. In addition, coke *does* increase concentration, as long as the user focuses on simple tasks or subjects. But any sense of increased competence beyond these limited effects are illusory.

- Sleeplessness. As a stimulant, cocaine reduces the need for sleep. In higher doses, it can lead to chronic insomnia.

- Heightened self-awareness. Cocaine users report that they feel more "in touch" with themselves when they use the drug. At its most extreme, this feeling can lead to insomnia.

- Altered sexual feelings. In low doses, cocaine enhances sexual excitement and performance. At higher doses or with chronic use, cocaine diminishes or replaces the desire for sex. The eventual result may be impotence or frigidity to the extent that not even cocaine can provide sexual pleasure.

- Reduced sense of humor. Users report that cocaine reduces the appreciation of jokes and the desire to laugh.

- Less involvement with the real world. Besides neglecting personal hygiene, chronic cocaine users become withdrawn from school, work, and social interaction.

- Perceptual changes. Hallucinations, distortion, and the sense that colors are brighter than normal are all common reactions to cocaine use. Distant objects may seem close by. Footsteps may be heard when no one is there. Users may experience itching, discomfort, a feeling of electricity passing through the body or of bugs crawling on the skin. Other sensations may include a sense that the arms and legs have grown longer, feelings of lightness, out-of-body experiences, or a sense of flying.

- Compulsive behavior. Users may perform the same tasks over and over again without any awareness of it. They may, for example, grind their teeth or constantly make chewing motions. As mentioned before, it's common to straighten up a room or desktop, wash dishes, or clean the stove or refrigerator continually.

- Addiction. For reasons I've already mentioned, cocaine—and especially crack—are incredibly addicting. In one study, 85 percent of users said they could not turn down cocaine if it were offered to them; 63 percent said they thought about the drug "continuously." More than 75 percent said it was preferable to grooming, friends, family, food, and sex. Three-quarters of these users believed themselves to be addicted, and 80 percent believed that cocaine was as physically addicting as any drug.

COCAINE'S EFFECTS ON THE BODY

Cocaine doesn't just play havoc with the brain; it ultimately affects all of the body's systems. These effects occur whether cocaine is sniffed, smoked, or injected, but the time span varies according to the method of use.

Cocaine's *physiologic* effects begin about five minutes after initial use when sniffed and can last up to one hour. The duration of the high itself is in direct proportion to the length of the route to the brain: the faster the cocaine reaches the brain, the sooner the effects subside. The cocaine sniffer's euphoria may be milder, but it lasts longer. Crack smokers experience a brief, but very intense, high.

The *side effects* of cocaine are often considered to be temporary and harmless. But in fact they can precipitate a trip to the emergency room—or to the morgue. Here's a list of side effects (the ones followed by an asterisk are identical to signs of a cocaine overdose, and anyone showing these signs needs to be observed by a physician for other signs of overdose):

- rapid pulse rate
- elevated blood pressure
- increased breathing rate
- sweating
- raised body temperature
- nausea, vomiting, abdominal pain*
- dry mouth
- dilated eye pupils*
- headache*
- tightening of muscles, including those controlling bowel movements
- urge to defecate, urinate, or belch
- slowdown of digestion and loss of appetite

- elevated blood sugar levels
- vitamin, mineral, and amino acid deficiency with continued cocaine use

As these effects dissipate, blood pressure and respiration often drop below normal levels, contributing to withdrawal symptoms and the craving for more of the drug.

Cocaine's physiologic devastation can linger well beyond the time when the drug is used. Studies at Fair Oaks Hospital, for example, have shown that use of the drug leads to severe vitamin deficiencies. One study showed that 73 percent of cocaine-abusing patients had deficiencies in at least one vitamin—most frequently B_6, B_1, and C. Cocaine causes most users to lose interest in food, which often leads to malnutrition.

Chronic cocaine users develop many diseases that are directly related to their drug use. For example, injected cocaine has been linked to inflammation of the liver (hepatitis) and of the heart lining (endocarditis). And chronic cocaine sniffers are familiar with the cocaine "freeze"—numbing of nasal passages, throat, and palate—which is linked to the anesthetic action of the drug. Constriction of the mucous membranes often creates a "rebound effect" in the blood vessels of the nose, causing congestion, sneezing, and head-cold symptoms. Chronic runny noses, nosebleeds, burns, sores, and upper respiratory infections are common.

Finally, chronic cocaine sniffers may suffer *septal necrosis*—that is, destruction of the mucous membranes and cartilage that separate the two nostrils. This condition, which is rare, can be repaired surgically.

Smoking crack bypasses many of the relatively mild symptoms that snorting cocaine causes. Users are at much greater risk for systemwide reactions, which can be far more severe and which are responsible for the overdoses and fatalities reported by hospital emergency rooms.

Most seriously affected are the respiratory, cardiovascular, and central nervous systems. Normally, these three systems work together to keep body functions in balance. Cocaine attacks each of them differently.

How much damage these systems suffer depends on the dose, the length of time that cocaine is used, and the purity of the drug when it is smoked or sniffed. We've already seen the effects that cocaine has on the nervous system. Below are some of the ways it affects the other two systems.

The Effects of Cocaine on the Respiratory System

- Tracheitis and chronic bronchitis (that is, inflammation of the trachea and bronchi, respectively)
- Hoarseness or even complete loss of voice
- Chronic heavy coughing and wheezing
- Coughs producing mucous, pus, blood, and in freebase smokers, a tarry residue

The Effects of Cocaine on the Cardiovascular System

While most cocaine sniffers suffer mild cardiovascular symptoms, crack smokers can experience stronger reactions, including the following:

- Irregular heart contractions and extremely rapid heart rate
- Increased blood pressure, which can "spike" so rapidly that it may lead to hemorrhage or congestive heart failure
- Chest pain from blood vessels around the heart

More serious cardiovascular effects include:

- Ashen gray skin, a sign of poorly oxygenated blood
- Overall failure of circulation (shock)
- Heart attack, damage to the heart muscle
- Death, caused by total heart failure

Coke's Effects on Other Conditions

Cocaine can also aggravate existing medical conditions including the following:

- Pregnancy and nursing. The direct effects of cocaine on a developing fetus aren't known. There are reports of cocaine use being associated with a higher rate of spontaneous miscarriage. Since cocaine use can lead to malnutrition of the mother, the unborn child is at the very least likely to be undernourished. Cocaine passes across the placenta, which causes a newborn baby to undergo withdrawal symptoms. The jitteriness and irritability of an addicted newborn is a heartrending sight. Cocaine is secreted in breast milk, and, for the reasons above, the breast milk of a coke user will probably be deficient in vitamins, minerals, and other substances vital to a nursing infant.

- Bronchitis and upper respiratory infections. Smoking crack can cause constant irritation of the breathing passages and increase the risk of infection by bacteria and viruses.

- Asthma. Shortness of breath and general breathing difficulties caused by smoking crack, together with anxiety reactions to the drug, can trigger asthma attacks.

- Anxiety. Generalized fears can escalate to the point where hospitalization is required.

- Depression. The more intense the cocaine high, the deeper the depression that follows. Hence, crack causes intense bouts of depression.

- Poor circulation. Coke's ability to constrict blood vessels aggravates circulatory problems.

- Heart problems. The same effect can decrease blood flow to the heart, causing angina or heart attacks. In addition, the drug can disrupt the heart's electrical system, causing heart attacks even in apparently healthy people.

- Epilepsy or seizures. Cocaine can cause seizures, and people suffering from seizure disorders have an increased danger of seizures from cocaine.

- Diabetes. Because cocaine increases blood sugar levels, it is especially dangerous for people with diabetes.

Serious Adverse Effects of Cocaine

Chronic use of crack and cocaine often leads to one or more serious adverse effects, most requiring medical attention and some of them potentially life-threatening:

- Severe digestive disorders. Erratic eating patterns and inadequate nutrition can result in chronic digestive problems.

- Dehydration. With loss of appetite comes loss of thirst, which can severely dehydrate the body.

- Anorexia. Permanent damage to the body's systems and lowered resistance to disease result from cocaine's appetite-suppressant properties. Death by malnutrition can occur.

- Hallucinations. Auditory and visual hallucinations usually accompany chronic cocaine use and may be signs of an overdose.

- "Impossible" overdose. A few people cannot metabolize cocaine, and even small doses remain in their bodies for a long time. A history of breathing problems under general anesthesia or after use of the muscle relaxant Anectine indicates the potential for a cocaine "overdose" after limited cocaine use.

MYTHS ABOUT CRACK

Over the years drugs like marijuana and LSD have been so mythologized that they have created a kind of folklore around them. Books featuring effects of marijuana and psychedelic drugs have been staples of literature for decades. Now crack seems to be developing its own misleading legends that help market the drug to inexperienced and vulnerable victims.

Myth: Crack is a cheap, purer form of cocaine.

Reality: Crack is neither pure nor cheap. If the cocaine that is used to make crack is cut with impurities before it's made, those impurities will remain in the freed base, often in a more intense state. If the cocaine powder is cut with a dangerous substance such as the local anesthetics lidocaine, benzocaine, or procaine, or more dangerous stimulants like amphetamine, phenylpropanolamine, and ephedrine, they will be left when the extraction of the cocaine base is complete. Often, these cuts are left in dangerous amounts, resulting in life-threatening reactions as the crack smoke rapidly enters the brain. The effect of the cuts with the powerful freed cocaine base can threaten the heart rhythm, blood pressure, and other important central nervous system functions.

Crack is more expensive than cocaine powder. Even though it is sold in inexpensive quantities, the price per gram is almost double that of cocaine powder. A $10 rock of crack usually weighs about 100 milligrams, which translates to $100 per gram. Further, since crack encourages its own taking, the user rarely stops until his entire bankroll is used up. Crack is by far a more expensive drug to use, not a cheaper one.

Myth: Crack is the ultimate "fun" drug.

Reality: Crack, unlike cocaine powder, is not associated with partying, disco dancing, and rock music. Crack's rush is so intense that most people want to use it quietly and in private, which has given rise to crack houses located in apartments or other protected environments. Crack use is rarely recreational. It usually occurs in binges lasting until the user or his money is exhausted.

Myth: Crack is an inner-city problem.

Reality: Many people think that crack use is limited to poor, urban teenagers. This myth has been reinforced by recent TV specials. However, our 800-COCAINE data indicates that crack use cuts across all segments of the population, ignoring economic, social, or ethnic restraints. The most common profile of a crack user is an adult male, aged twenty to thirty. While adolescents are not yet the major user group, they are the most vulnerable. It also seems from anecdotal observation that crack users are often those who want to experience the most intense events, while other drug abusers may be frightened by its power.

Myth: Crack users are easy to identify.

Reality: Crack use, as distinct from other cocaine use, can't be identified by urine tests. It will simply be identified as cocaine. And there's no single sign of crack use in a medical test that separates it from cocaine powder use. The most reliable methods of detecting cocaine use are through other physiologic symptoms such as respiratory changes or behavioral actions.

THE GOOD NEWS

There is one piece of good news about cocaine addiction: The cycle *can* be broken. But it's not easy, and it's almost impossible to do on your own. A little later on, we'll look at how people can get off cocaine and stay off after they stop. But before we do, there are some people I want you to meet.

· 3 ·

Kids on Crack

The best way I know to show you how crack affects kids is to let you read their stories. Not long ago, I sat down with five teenagers who are recovering from years of drug addiction. I asked them to talk about what life was like for them before they got into treatment. To protect their privacy, I've changed their names and some other details, but their stories are all very real.

The things they told me may send shivers down your spine. But what's even scarier is that these are not disadvantaged kids from the inner city; they're ordinary teenagers from affluent suburban neighborhoods. I've heard similar accounts from many other kids. What happened to them could and does happen to anyone anywhere.

These are excerpts from an interview with teenage patients at Fair Oaks Hospital. If you'd never met them before, you'd think they were simply a bunch of teenage kids, perhaps getting together to work on a school project.

Gary is a tall, outgoing sixteen-year-old, talkative and quick to smile.

Dennis is a year older, and has a dark and quiet look. He chooses his words carefully, and you get the feeling that he keeps a lot inside.

Davy, red-haired, with a stocky frame and fading acne scars, looks and talks like the typical kid next door.

Carol is an attractive girl of sixteen. She's nervous and tends to bite her nails while she's talking.

Rich is different from the other four. He's seventeen, but he has the deep voice and five-o'clock shadow of someone who's much older. There's something in the way he acts and talks, too, that sets him apart from the other kids. At the beginning of the session, he settles into the chair opposite mine, and the kids to left and right move their chairs away a little—as if they're afraid of him.

In the months that the group has been in treatment, these five teenagers have come to know one another better than anyone ever knew them in their lives. And yet they're not exactly friends. Their bond is more like that shared by survivors of a war. In a sense, they *are* survivors of battles that my colleagues and I know only secondhand.

Most of our meetings are held in a sunny conference room at the hospital; on warm days, we may sit outside under the trees. And yet when the kids begin to talk, you can see from their eyes that the pleasant surroundings are far away. They are reliving a life of endless nights in shuttered rooms, of furtive street-corner meetings where vast sums of money change hands, of roller-coaster rides from the heights of euphoria to the depths of despair.

None of them originally came to the hospital of his own free will—in fact, few of them came under their own power. Many of our teenage patients arrive like Rich did—dirty, emaciated, and seemingly unaware of where he was or why. Others, like Gary, are openly hostile at first to the idea of treatment and only want to get back to their old ways and friends. Some, like Carol, quickly learn to trust us and to cooperate with us.

Our experience tells us that some of these kids may go back to drugs after they leave here. For many, the battle against drug use will be a constant and lifelong struggle. But with hard work and support from others, these kids can put their lives back together. I'm proud of all of them and of how far they've come.

Let's start with you telling us your name, your age, and what your parents do for a living.

GARY: My name's Gary. My father's a carpenter, my mother's a teacher. I'm sixteen.

DENNIS: My name's Dennis. My mom's an office supervisor and I'm seventeen.

DAVY: My name's Davy. My mother's a nurse, my father's a fireman, a bartender, and an alcoholic.

RICH: My name's Rich. I'm seventeen. My father's an economist and my mother teaches dance.

CAROL: My name is Carol. I'm sixteen. My mother and father are in communications.

How old were each of you when you first started using any drugs?
GARY: Nine.

What did you start with, Gary?
GARY: Reefer.[1]
DENNIS: I'd say about thirteen.
DAVY: Thirteen, fourteen. I started with alcohol.
DENNIS: Alcohol.
RICH: Nine. With alcohol.
CAROL: Ten, with alcohol.

Okay. Now, can you give me a list of all the drugs you've used?
Gary?
GARY: Pot. Coke. Crack. Mescaline. Acid. Speed. Crystal meth. Smack. Base. Dust.[2] Sometimes alcohol.

DENNIS: Alcohol. Pot. Coke. Mescaline. LSD. Amyl nitrate.[3] Speed and Valium.

DAVY: Coke. Crack. Reefer. Alcohol. Acid. Mescaline. Mushrooms. Ecstasy.[4] Speed. Smack.

---

1. Marijuana.
2. Pot is slang for marijuana. *Mescaline* and *acid* (LSD) are hallucinogens. *Speed* and *crystal meth* are amphetamines. *Smack* is heroin. *Base* is freebase cocaine. *Dust* is angel dust (PCP), a synthetic hallucinogen that is sometimes referred to—erroneously—as THC. (Real THC is the active ingredient in marijuana and hashish; it is difficult to make and is unavailable on the street.)
3. *Amyl nitrate* is a heart medication that is chemically related to nitroglycerin; when inhaled, it produces a brief but powerful "rush."
4. Psilocybin *mushrooms* contain a hallucinogenic substance that is similar to, but less potent than, LSD. *Ecstasy* is a "designer" drug, recently outlawed, that is chemically similar to amphetamines.

RICH: Alcohol. Pot. Ludes [Quaaludes]. Valium. Speed. Ups [amphetamines]. Downs [barbiturates]. Acid. Mesc [mescaline]. Crack. Base. Dust. That's about it.

CAROL: Alcohol. Pot. Cocaine. Mescaline. Valium. Crack.

What were you using just before you came in here?
DAVY: Freebase.[5]

And that's how you ended up here?
DAVY: See, I'd had a party, spent twenty-five hundred dollars, and I was too high and I took twenty-six Valiums.

Where did you get twenty-five hundred dollars?
DAVY: I was working. I saved up about a year and a half, two years.

And you spent that much money over what period of time?
DAVY: I spent that in—well, I had done it in a pipe in three days.

Three days.
DAVY: With a bunch of friends.

You just threw a party for everybody? And you supplied the free-base?
DAVY: Well, first I had a couple of friends over, then they would leave, and bring friends over a couple hours later, and it just got really big.

This was in your parents' home?
DAVY: Um-hm. In the basement.

Where were they?
DAVY: Upstairs.

They knew about it?
DAVY: No. They knew I was downstairs, though.

---

5. Freebase, like crack, is a smokable form of cocaine. See chapter two.

So they just left you alone?
DAVY: They didn't know I was really getting high. They thought that I was having friends over and the music was going.

For three days?
DAVY: Yeah.

Tell me, what was the crack high like?
DAVY: So good I needed more.
CAROL: The high from it was so—such a rush, you know—it was different.

Did you like it?
CAROL: I liked it but it scared me.
GARY: The high was like stronger and more rushier.

Speeds you more?
GARY: Yeah. I loved it.

When you say that, what do you mean?
GARY: Loved it? That was my girlfriend, my mother, my father, my family—it was everything in my life.

What do you mean by that?
GARY: It means I associated with that pipe twenty hours a day.

So you were in love with your pipe and everything else—
GARY: —was shut out.

Family? Girlfriend? Did you have a girlfriend at the time?
GARY: Yeah.

What happened to her?
GARY: I was going with her in November, and January first we broke up.

Because of your drug use?
GARY: Yeah. Because I didn't want to go out, I just wanted to sit around and smoke.

Rich?

RICH: I loved it. It was my self-esteem.

What do you mean?

RICH: During the day I lived for it. And towards the end, I'd wake up in the morning, and the first thing I'd do was take a hit. I wouldn't get out of bed till I got a hit.

What's the most vials you've done in a binge?

RICH: Twenty-three, twenty-four. Somewhere in the twenties.

Why did you stop there?

RICH: Because I was speeding so much I sort of had a heart attack.

What do you mean? Chest pains?

RICH: Very bad. I had to lay in bed for a weekend.

Did you see a doctor about it?

RICH: No.

What was the chest pain like? Did it really feel like you were having a heart attack?

RICH: It felt like a knife going right through my heart and I couldn't lean forward or lean back. I just had to lay flat.

How long did that last?

RICH: Two days.

Two days? With that kind of pain?

RICH: I got it Saturday morning and I had it till about Monday, Sunday night.

How much were you doing before you came in here? Davy?

DAVY: Before I came here I was mainly using alcohol every night, a six [pack] or two a night, smoking pot almost every night—about an eighth of an ounce or so a night—and a lot of cocaine.

How much cocaine were you doing?

DAVY: There were splurges. Some weeks I'd do only an eighth of a gram all night. I had one big splurge where I took close to twenty grams with a couple friends in one night. And with that I was taking acid and mescaline.

Where would you get the money for twenty grams of coke?

DAVY: I stole the money.

What did you steal?

DAVY: Checks, from my mom's bank account, my grandmother's bank account. Money from work.

Didn't they miss the money? I mean your family?

DAVY: My family missed it and that's how everything really mounted up.

So that's how they really began to know that something was wrong.

DAVY: They could see something was going on.

What's the most money you've stolen at one time?

DAVY: At one time? I stole maybe five, six hundred dollars in cash and merchandise from a store.

How about from your parents? What was the most you would take out of the bank account?

DAVY: Four hundred.

Rich? What were you using just before you came in?

RICH: Crack, coke, and alcohol.

How much?

RICH: I was doing one to two grams a night and one to two hundred dollars of base or two hundred dollars of crack. And anywhere from a six pack to a case of beer or a quart of scotch.

You were doing one to two hundred dollars of crack a day? How many vials[6] would you be doing in a day?

RICH: It depends. If I got the ten-dollar bottles, I'd be doing anywhere from twenty to thirty.

CAROL: Before I came in I was doing alcohol, pot, and cocaine. I guess in the end I was using about two quarts of beer a day. And I'd do coke too—some days might be better than other days. There'd be days when I would do maybe an eighth [of a gram], while on a good day—in a two-day period—I did eighteen grams of coke.

Alone or with friends?

CAROL: Alone, by myself. At other times it was with friends.

Where would you get the money for that?

CAROL: I was dealing at the time and then I would steal from my mother, and I would pawn my jewelry sometimes.

Because you're talking about well over a thousand dollars. How would you steal that?

CAROL: The most I've ever stolen from my mother is about four hundred dollars. And the rest came from dealing.

How would you steal four hundred dollars from your mom?

CAROL: It wouldn't be in just one day. It would be over a period of a couple days or so.

How many of you dealt? All of you? Okay. And were you dealing other drugs, or crack or coke or—

DAVY: I dealt everything.

SEVERAL VOICES: Acid. Ecstasy. Valium.

Okay. When did each of you start doing crack and how much were you using? What was it like? Just tell me a little bit about the whole crack thing.

GARY: I started in '84. I was cooking it—

6. Crack is sold in small bottles or vials.

You're talking about freebase.

GARY: Yeah. But later on when the crack thing started getting big on the street, I'd just be too bugged out to cook [freebase], so I would buy crack.[7]

When did you start to switch over from your own freebasing to crack?

GARY: Last year, before Christmas.

Why did you switch over?

GARY: Well, I didn't really switch over. But if it was like at three o'clock in the morning when I was really bugging out and I didn't want to cook—just wanted to do more—I would just go down and buy crack—

So it was easier?

GARY: Yeah.

RICH: I started doing crack in the middle of April.

How did you get into crack?

RICH: My friend said he wanted to get crack and I said I'd try it. And I tried it and liked it, and I knew I would get crazy with the stuff.

Why?

RICH: Because every other drug I do I—

—You get crazy.

RICH: —can't do just one. Like I take six hits of mescaline. I can't smoke one joint, I have to smoke ten joints. So I started doing crack and I'd be fine for the day if I didn't touch it. But if I had one hit, from the time I had that hit to the time I went to bed I couldn't stop.

---

7. Freebase is "cooked" with volatile chemicals before it is smoked—a complicated and dangerous process. (Comedian Richard Pryor nearly died from an explosion while cooking freebase.) One of the appeals of crack is that it gives the intense high of freebase without the need to cook it.

So if you stayed away from it, you were okay, but once you used it—

RICH: I couldn't stop for the rest of the day.

Where were your parents during all of your drug use? Davy, you mentioned you had a party and they were upstairs. How much did your parents know about your drug use?

DAVY: My mother was in denial the whole time. My father kept telling her two years ago when they got married that I was on drugs. But she didn't want to believe it.

So he saw it and she denied it, and so she just ignored it when you were partying?

DAVY: It was more like she couldn't do nothing about it because I was out for three, four—one time I was out for two weeks, out of the house—

Without her knowing where you were?

DAVY: Yeah.

They didn't do anything about that?

DAVY: Yeah. They called the cops. I live in a small town, and if I don't want to be found, I'm not going to get found.

How about the rest of you? Where were your parents?

RICH: My parents knew I was getting high because I told them in November last year that I had a problem with mesc and pot and alcohol. And I told them I'd stop, and they thought I stopped.

Did you try to stop?

RICH: I lasted two days.

Two days. How about the rest of you? Did you ever try to stop drugs?

DENNIS: Every day.

Every day you tried to stop?

DENNIS: I would say to myself, "This is the last time."

How long would it last? A day?

DENNIS: Not even.

GARY: My parents were at home during my drug use.

Did any of your parents know you were doing drugs?

RICH: When I told them in November. That's when they found out I was doing drugs.

And they had no idea before you told them.

RICH: When I used to come home I'd stumble and everything, and my mother would say, "What's wrong with you?" I'd say I had too much beer. Alcohol's my best excuse.

So you could just blame everything on alcohol. And that was okay?

RICH: Yeah. And I'd go home at night and I'd be on mesc or acid and I'd just sit down in my living room and talk to them.

And they wouldn't notice that you were high or—

RICH: They'd say something like, "What's the matter?" I'd say I was drunk.

DENNIS: Well, at first I couldn't really hide it—you know, my eyes would get red and all that stuff. Then after a while I could hide it from her. Like I'd look into a light for a couple seconds so my pupils would be really small.

What were some of the craziest things you've done on crack?

GARY: I stabbed somebody in the arm for a hit.

What happened?

GARY: We were sitting at a table and I put a big rock in and this other guy kept smoking and smoking. There was enough for four people and he kept smoking. So I said, "Gimme it, gimme it, give me the pipe, give me the pipe." And he wouldn't. I stabbed him in the arm. I got so nervous I ran out of the house and haven't seen the kid since.

DAVY: Set my house off. It looked like we got robbed.

What do you mean? How did you do that?

DAVY: I destroyed the place. Wrecked it.

Why?
DAVY: I wrecked it, took the color TV, took the stereo systems.

The whole house? Or just—
DAVY: The whole house.

What did you get away with?
DAVY: TV, stereo—three stereo systems—diamond rings, diamond necklaces, anything that was valuable was gone, out of the house and into the back of the car.

Where did you take it?
DAVY: Down to the Bronx.

To the Bronx. And just sold it to a store—
DAVY: The color TV I took to the Bronx and the stereo and the rings and stuff went to Newark.

To a jeweler's?
DAVY: No, to a dealer over there.

Okay, how about the rest of you?
CAROL: I came home one night really high and I didn't have any more money. My mother wasn't home and I had left my key in the house and I couldn't find it, so I threw a rock through the front-door window and opened the door. And I took all my brother's money that was sitting in his room, I took my brother's radio and left, and I left the door like that. My mom came home before I did, and when I eventually came home that night she asked me about it. And I told her I didn't know anything about it.

Did you ever do anything sexually for drugs? Or while you were high?
CAROL: Guys always tried to buy you like that, so most of the time what I would do is go get high with them and tell them I'd meet them somewhere, and I'd take off. And then with the next guy I'd do the same thing.
RICH: I was downtown one night with a friend. We went to a prostitute and we paid her—did things with her. Then she asked

me to drive her to a friend's house. As I was driving, we turned a corner really fast and flew onto a side street where my friend pulled her head back and cut her neck open.

Say that again!
RICH: He was in the back seat, she was in the front seat next to me.

Why did you do that?
RICH: Because she had money on her and we didn't. I was high. It turned out to be only $20.

You think maybe you killed her?
RICH: Yeah. I don't want to think about it.

What's the worst thing about crack for each of you?
RICH: Fiending.

What do you mean by fiending?
RICH: After you've done all you can—put all your money out and done all you can do and start coming down, you don't have that rush no more—you'll do anything for anyone to get it. You'll go anywhere and do anything.

Like what?
RICH: Like if I go out for a night and have coke and pick up a girl, I expect something from the girl at the end of the night. When I was on the bottom with crack and I couldn't think or anything, there was a guy who offered me what I wanted—crack—but he expected something from me, homosexually. And I didn't care.

Would you ever do it?
RICH: I did it.

Is that the fiending? What do you mean by fiending?
GARY: Just—I need more and I'm going to do anything to get it.
DAVY: It's a devil coming out of you. My last bout before I went to the hospital, my mother was crying, and I said, "Ma, what's happening to me? I think a devil took over my body."

*Is there anything that could have been done to help you before you
came into treatment? I mean, is there anything that you can tell
parents or anything that you might have listened to? I'm sure most
of you had drug programs in school, you heard it on the news—*

GARY: I've been to a lot of schools and not one had a drug program.

None had a drug program?

CAROL: Mine did.

Did you listen to it?

RICH: My drug counselor begged me to go to rehab from November to April sixteenth.

And what did you do?

RICH: I said, "I don't have a drug problem; I just like to get high."

DENNIS: I was in two or three different programs before I came
out here. But I'd go in a program, and as soon as I was out I'd go get
high.

GARY: There's nothing that you can do. Your parents have to do it
all and they have to put you here.

What do you mean, Gary?

GARY: In my case I always said I didn't have a drug problem.

*So what you're saying is that there's nothing people can do except
get you into treatment.*

SEVERAL VOICES: That's the only thing.

CAROL: But before it goes this far, the kids aren't listening. Because I know I didn't listen in the school when they had all the
programs, all the people that had come in. Parents need to start
listening, to watch, maybe, and to learn a lot more than they're
learning.

Is there anything that you could say to other kids?

DAVY: They wouldn't listen.

GARY: My mother used to bring the kids that OD'd at school to
the hospital, kids with drug problems, and I was around these kids
that had all these problems and I didn't listen, man.

Were any of you ever around recovering kids?
SEVERAL VOICES: Yeah.

What was your reaction to them? Did you just ignore them and think they were—
RICH: I'd say, "Let's smoke a joint."

So you tried to tease them back into doing drugs.
CAROL: I just ignored them. Didn't think twice about it.
RICH: I remember when the commercials for crack first came on TV—it must have been four-thirty, five in the morning. I'd be at this girl's house, and I'd sit there and as the commercial said, "Don't do crack," I'd be sitting there with a crack pipe in my mouth.

How many of you think you're winning the battle against drugs? In your own life.
GARY: I got it.
DENNIS: I'm working.
RICH: I'm ready to go home.

What is it that's really helped you? In the battle. I mean, what works?
GARY: Ken [a counselor].

What works about him?
GARY: He gets you to think, and not like a drug addict.

What do you mean?
CAROL: He really makes you think, but makes you think clear— you know, reality and not this fantasy world most of us have lived in.

The drug world is a fantasy world. It really is, isn't it?
GARY: A sick, sick world.
DENNIS: It also makes you realize that you are a drug addict.

Did any of you think you were a drug addict before you came in here?
SEVERAL VOICES: I knew I was. Um-hm. Yeah.

CAROL: Well, I didn't say it, but—

GARY: I liked it.

DENNIS: I didn't.

You didn't think you were an addict?

DENNIS: No, not at all. Even when I went into the outpatient program.

CAROL: I didn't think about it. Didn't think about ever not doing it.

GARY: I said, "Hey, when I'm twenty years old I'll stop."

RICH: I thought I was going to die. So when I started smoking pot, I said, "This is what I do now, and it's how I'm going to die." I thought there was nothing left to help me.

Did part of you want to die?

RICH: Yeah.

And the drugs were sort of a slow way to do it?

RICH: Yeah.

DAVY: I was within hours of death. I came in—I OD'd on Valium and the doctors kept telling me I wasn't normal; twenty-six Valiums kill a normal person.

That was what got you in here?

DAVY: Otherwise I would have run from here.

Some of you guys have talked about when you finish treatment, going to a concert with your Crackbusters T-shirts. What's important about that?

GARY: I want to tell them that I don't want to smoke crack.

RICH: It says you can have a good time without drugs. Because I had to learn that and I did. That was the hardest thing to learn.

That's the hardest thing—that you can still have fun and have a good time without drugs.

GARY: I'm leaving this afternoon. I'm leaving this hospital, and I have come such a long way.

What are you thinking about as you leave this afternoon?

GARY: All the things that I'm going to do straight. And all the people I'm going to meet that are straight.

In your aftercare?

GARY: In my aftercare and my meetings.

So you're looking forward to recovery?

GARY: I am.

· 4 ·

Understanding Adult and Teen Addiction

The frightening dialogue you've just read is from a real interview session with teens who are recovering from drug addiction. They're not moral degenerates. They were not reared in deprived environments. They are otherwise normal teenagers who suffer from a common widespread disease: addiction. One reason that we have failed to understand addiction is that we have allowed myth to obscure fact about drug abuse. Myths are hard to destroy, but to reduce drug abuse and to eliminate the threat of drugs like crack, we must try. One important myth to dispel is that teenagers are the only ones vulnerable to drugs like crack. Read this typical case described by my colleague Dr. Mark Gold in his book, *800-CO-CAINE*.[1]

Just thirty-two, Linda C. was the woman of the eighties with everything going for her. She was an attractive redhead who had climbed up the corporate ladder to a high-level executive position in a major publishing house. She lunched at The Four Seasons with well-known authors and edited number-one bestsellers. Her income allowed her a lifestyle of weekend vacation houses, de-

---

signer clothing, and an apartment with a dazzling view of Central Park. Linda expected that she would one day head her publishing house, and she considered her life a model for young women just entering the work force.

On one of her weekends in the Hamptons, she met a stockbroker whom she believed was everything she'd always wanted. He was well-to-do, charming, polite, and looking for the same type of relationship she wanted. Within a few months their relationship was so solid that Linda decided to let him move into her apartment.

Linda had used drugs before she met her boyfriend. In fact, she had experimented with LSD, marijuana, and other drugs in her twenties. Her drug use, though, was casual and actually she preferred a good, expensive bottle of wine to drugs. If she had any problem with drugs, she said it was "getting drunk one time too many." She did not feel she was chemically dependent.

Her boyfriend had not told her everything, though. He had not mentioned that most of his income came from his cocaine dealing rather than his stockbroker's job. By the time she'd figured out the extent of his drug dealing, he'd also introduced her to crack. Ironically, the drug initially helped cement their relationship. She thought it provided a good aphrodisiac. "The sex was pretty good at first," she said.

Since she now had a virtually unlimited supply—and free—she found that she was using it regularly every weekend. Then, within three months, every night.

"I became a classic clock watcher," Linda remembers. "Although I'd never use it during the day, for fear it would interfere with my work, when the clock hit five, I was out the door. I'd bolt for home without stopping. The cravings for the crack were that intense."

It wasn't long before Linda's crack smoking took over her days, too. "All my work patterns were affected. Where I'd been the model of a professional—calm, reasoned, and quick—I became short-tempered and paranoid," Linda recalls. "I lost interest in my friends and in any after-work social activities."

Linda's coworkers and her boss quickly noticed the change. But her boss, who knew little about drugs but a lot about Linda, felt that her behavior was linked to her new romantic relationship or perhaps alcohol use. There had been an ugly incident at lunch the week before, when Linda had gotten drunk at an editorial "bull session" held at a local restaurant.

While Linda denied that she had any problems at all to her boss and friends at work, she knew that her life was unraveling. She later recalled that at this point she actually had no idea how much crack she was using since it was always around the apartment. Then one night she found herself faced with a dilemma she simply couldn't solve.

Her boss had insisted that she go to a sales conference in the Bahamas. It meant she'd be away from her source of drugs for at least a week. And it also meant that she'd have to risk traveling abroad with her own drug supply, a risk she didn't want to take. She had given her boss virtually every excuse she could muster to avoid the trip, but nothing had worked. She was trapped and she felt helpless. As she stared out her window, down at the Park, it occurred to her that she was at the end of the line.

The answer was obvious. Jump.

She'd already lost her career—she was on the verge of being fired and certainly would be if she failed to show up for the sales conference. Her personal life was nonexistent. Every day revolved around crack. She didn't dare try to alter her relationship or she'd lose her crack supply.

Linda turned away from the window and looked in the mirror. She felt only one emotion—fear. She had managed in a short three months to scare herself almost to death. She called my colleague Dr. Arnold Washton who had successfully treated a friend and asked if she could commit herself to Regent Hospital.

Linda's story, like all the other shocking stories, demonstrates that addiction is a process. It's part of a very broad picture we call "chemical dependency." Even though these cases show that drugs like crack have a major impact on an adult's or teenager's value system, they do not indicate that chemical dependency is a moral problem.

Addiction is a disease with moral consequences. We must approach it as we would any other disease process. We look at signs, symptoms, causes, the course of the illness, and finally treatment forms that will be most helpful to the eventual recovery of the person.

WHAT ARE THE EFFECTS OF DRUG ABUSE?

Even before the crack epidemic began, we'd reached some conclusions about the nature of drug abuse and cocaine addiction that changed how we view patients. We've even redefined the concept of drug abuse. We also learned about the subject and confirmed our theories by carefully examining the information we received from the 800-COCAINE helpline over the past three years. Not surprisingly, we've learned that most people are very misinformed about drug actions and effects. We have also learned that old definitions of addiction mean very little in the context of powerful drugs like crack and of recent research on cocaine and other drugs.

The quickest way to understand the power of drugs and what has happened to the people we've described in this book is to see what is involved in the process of addiction that results from drug abuse.

Drug abuse leads to a state of chemical dependency—a developing reliance on drugs that alter moods to achieve pleasure and happiness. When this dependency becomes stronger, we often refer to it as "addiction." The addictive disease process has three main factors. In fact, you can look at it in terms of an equation:

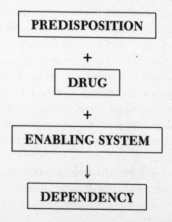

Consider each part of this equation.

Predisposition to addiction has four possible sources: heredity, physiology, psychology, and socioculture. We've been able to determine these four factors after years of studying alcoholics. One of the reasons for using alcoholics for this research is that it has been easier to find people addicted to alcohol alone than addicted to any other single mood-altering drug.

Heredity: The evidence that heredity plays a role in addiction is borne out by studies of twins. Studies of identical twins (with the same genetic material) show that if one is addicted, there is a 54 percent chance the other will be. If a fraternal twin with half of the genetic material in common becomes addicted, there is a 28 percent chance. Both of these ratios are far higher than that of the general population. One way of determining how much of this is genetic rather than environmental is to look at adoption studies. Adoption studies show that sons of alcoholic fathers have a four to five times greater rate of alcoholism than the general population, regardless of whether they are raised by nonalcoholic foster parents or by their own biological and alcoholic parent.

The statistical evidence is overwhelming. Examine your own family history to see if there's a predisposition to addiction just as you would if a parent or grandparent had heart disease. It's vital to know all the health risks you may face.

Physiology: Similar twin studies also show that physiology can play a process in predisposition. Several enzymes connected with the breakdown of alcohol in alcoholics and nonalcoholics suggest that the biology or the nature of one's system plays a role in addiction. Brainwave studies in sons of alcoholics as opposed to nonalcoholics have confirmed some of these suspicions. Of course, we aren't sure yet whether the biological evidence is linked to environmental factors.

Psychology: Is there such thing as an addictive personality? Many people think so and use it as an excuse or rationalization for why they aren't addicted but their drug-using friends are. What is the truth?

For many years we searched for what would be an addictive personality. We looked for common factors such as low thresholds of frustration and impulse control, and general neurosis. We discovered that there is no single psychological characteristic—no common thread that links those who become addicted. Seemingly well-adjusted, "normal" people become addicted as do those who have obvious behavioral or emotional problems. (In chapter five this subject is discussed in relation to teenagers whose personality traits may play a role in the addictive process.)

Socioculture: While harder to demonstrate scientifically, there is some evidence that sociocultural factors contribute to the addictive process. These could include age, occupation, social class, and even religious affiliation.

The *Drug:* By now you've figured out that the road to chemical dependency is not a straight road. When the drug is introduced into the addiction equation, it becomes even more complex.

First, each drug affects different people differently. This is especially true of teenagers. Which drug, how much, potency of dosage, where it's obtained, and how it's used (alone or in combination) are all part of the effect of the drug in the chemical dependency equation.

Crack is a good example. As we've seen, its intense, rapid effect leads to a rapid dependency and addiction in almost anyone who uses it. Marijuana has a much slower effect and produces a longer buildup of physiological and psychological effects. Alcohol is yet another drug with a different biochemical effect and different sociocultural implications.

The *availability* of a drug is a major factor in the *drug* part of the equation. Obviously, the more crack that is available, the more cocaine that is available, the faster an addiction can occur. Many addicts report that the amount of drugs they could get their hands on was a definite factor in how fast or slowly their addiction developed. One study showed that an estimated 20 percent of GIs in Vietnam developed heroin addiction—a much higher incidence than usual. *But,* over 90 percent were able to beat that addiction once they returned from Vietnam.

The last part of the equation is the *Enabling System. Enabling is the people part of the equation.* It's the "attitudes" part of the equation, and wrong attitudes are often—in fact, almost always—present in addiction. Enablers are the people in your life who either ignore someone's drug use or unwittingly assist it. Because it is closely linked to teen drug abuse, we will focus on this in the next chapter. For the moment, though, let's dispel some more myths of drug abuse and addiction before we reach a definition of addiction that fits our equation.

WHAT KIND OF ADDICTION DO YOU HAVE: PHYSICAL OR PSYCHOLOGICAL?

One of the great myths about addiction is the misconception that it's "better" or less serious to have a "psychological" addiction than a "physical" addiction. For many years people thought this was an important distinction to make.

The fact is that this distinction is no longer clear. Physical addiction usually meant that there was the development of a *tolerance* to the drug and that stopping drug use led to a specific *withdrawal syndrome*. When you take most illegal drugs or most types of mood altering drugs, your body develops *tolerance*. This simply means that the dose you've been taking no longer does the job. You need more and more to get the same effect because your body has adjusted to the dose. Since drugs are typed by class, there is very little chance that you can avoid tolerance by switching to a similar drug. You will automatically become addicted to a drug of the same class if you are addicted to another. For example, if you are addicted to benzodiazepines like Valium, you will become addicted to other sedatives like alcohol. This tolerance extends even further. If you are addicted to any class of mood altering drugs, for example cocaine, you are also likely to become addicted to any other, like alcohol, that you may try.

Another sign of physical addiction is the presence of a *withdrawal syndrome* when the drug is discontinued. Withdrawal usually appears soon after a drug is stopped and is usually specific to each drug. As we've described in chapter two, abrupt cessation of crack causes cravings due to neurotransmitter depletion. Abruptly stopping alcohol can cause a wide variety of effects—tremors, weakness, increased heart rate, and delirium tremens (DTs). In the past, withdrawal effects were primarily associated with opiates such as heroin. "Junkie" movies showed a heroin addict sweating out his withdrawal, writhing in pain strapped to a hospital bed. But in fact most drugs, even marijuana or cocaine powder, have a physical withdrawal aspect when stopped abruptly.

SO, WHAT IS ADDICTION?

Until we learned more about how cocaine affected the brain, it was thought that it led to no real physical addiction—only a psychological one. We now know that is not true. And it is partially as a result of this information that we can say that the distinction between a physical and a psychological addiction is not very clear or helpful. We prefer to use a broader definition of addiction:

> **Addiction is an irresistible compulsion to use a drug at increasing dose and frequency even in the presence of serious physical or psychological side effects and the extreme disruption of the user's personal relationships and system of values.**

Addiction is simply compulsive use with loss of control in spite of adverse consequences.

This definition, when applied to excessive jogging, cigarette smoking, drinking, gambling, or even video games, helps you see that "being addicted" isn't an activity limited to illegal drugs. Interestingly, research has shown that some biologically predisposed addicts may also become food-addicted because similar physiologic mechanisms are triggered by overeating. Research at Fair Oaks Hospital in our Eating Disorders Center indicates that eating disorders like bulimia or anorexia may also be so-called autoaddictions.

If you understand addiction as defined above, then it's also easy to see why we say that it's a process:

Use . . . leads to . . . tolerance . . . leads to . . . abuse . . . leads to . . . chemical dependence and addiction.

This new definition dispels the myth of the weak-willed junkie, hooked after a single dose of crack.

Drug addicts are not moral failures but victims of a disease caused by a variety of biological, chemical, and sociological circumstances.

Another myth is that all drug addicts use drugs every day. This isn't true. Different addicts have different patterns of drug abuse. You may be able to control your addiction on certain days but not the amount you use on days that you take the drug. Once you begin using a drug, you'll use it until it's gone.

It's important to remember that this does not *make it all right* to start using a drug. You are never absolved of the responsibility of using an illegal drug; however, once you are using the drug and become dependent, the drug uses you. You have lost control. This is so even if there is a preceding illness, for instance, depression. The drug must be removed from the body system before treating the other problem. Often, an addict enters treatment in our hospital and has signs and symptoms of depression. If he is allowed to be drug free, the depression clears up in many of these people. However, sometimes, even after the drug is removed, there may still be a psychiatric illness that needs further treatment. The depression may have led them to taking drugs to feel better.

With this new understanding of the addictive process, we recognize that you need to seek help from a program that treats addiction as a "primary illness." By this we mean that even though the illness may stem from quite diverse physical/psychological origins, once the addiction has been grafted onto this pre-existing behavior and personality structure, it dominates the clinical picture and controls the behavior. This means that the drug addiction must be a major focus in treatment.

HOW IMPORTANT ARE "SOCIAL" FACTORS?

Lifestyle and attitude can influence the development of addiction. Lifestyle does *not* determine *who* becomes drug- or alcohol-dependent, although it can be part of the process that leads to the eventual development of an addictive disease.

Attitude may be influential because it can determine whether or not you ever try drugs. If you believe all mood altering drugs are bad then you may never be around people who use drugs. Unfortunately, community attitudes toward drugs have led to the epidemic we face today. Many people consider certain drugs socially acceptable.

Occupation is not usually involved in drug-use patterns. But if you work in an environment where drug use is common or even the norm, you may have more opportunity to abuse drugs. This doesn't mean you're a rock musician; plenty of Wall Street stockbrokers are coke or even crack addicts. Although attitudes are finally changing, in the past many in glamorous occupations like major league sports, high-pressure sales, film, and other professions tolerated drug use as "necessary" to get the job done.

More recently, drug use has spread into the industrial work force, and the effects can be seen on the assembly line and in critical industries like high-tech computer companies, air transportation, and even nuclear power plants.

Other triggers include *stress* and the *setting* (alcohol use in your home can be safe—on the road it may be fatal).

The *availability* and *price* of drugs may be related to your occupation or where you work or live, and may also affect your use of drugs. Today, crack or cocaine powder, marijuana, tobacco, alcohol, and prescription drugs are widely abused because they are everywhere. And their price is within reach of virtually everyone.

ARE YOU HOOKED?

How can you tell if you or someone close to you has a drug or alcohol problem? We have devised a short test for you to take, but before you do, here are a few other important aspects of addiction to keep in mind:

1. All drug and alcohol abusers have one thing in common—*denial*. Virtually everyone who has a problem with substance abuse says, "I don't have a problem. I can handle it." The more they are confronted with evidence of a problem, the more defensive they become.

2. Most people with untreated drug problems feel they "need the drug to function normally." This is another common symptom of a person whose drug/alcohol use is already out of control.

3. If you experience increased "craving" for the substance, you are in serious trouble. In chapter two we explained a little more about why you "crave" crack more and more from a physiologic standpoint. But if you need more of any substance each day just to feel normal—not even to feel high—you need help.

4. If you can identify any of these general symptoms *or* you have a family history of some sort of chemical dependency or addiction, you should seek treatment.

There are also physical, mental, behavioral, and social changes that indicate you may be in trouble with drugs. Look at the following list and see if you or someone you suspect is abusing drugs or alcohol displays any of the following symptoms. They can be indications that something is wrong. Their presence does not mean that someone is *definitely* suffering from addiction—because they may be symptoms of other disease—but they are signs and symptoms usually linked to drug abuse or addiction.

Physical and Mental Symptoms of Addiction

- increased or decreased tolerance for alcohol or drugs
- red face, red nose
- bumps and bruises (from falling, etc.)
- puffiness of face or extremities
- sudden vision difficulties
- swollen nasal membrane
- chest and heart problems including bronchitis, changed heart rhythms, heart failure
- enlarged liver
- frequent infections
- digestive problems
- lingering colds and flu
- high blood pressure
- signs of bad nutrition
- tremors
- blackouts
- changes in reflexes
- loss of coordination
- dizziness
- confusion and slow comprehension
- slurred speech
- memory loss
- anxiety or depression
- delirium
- hallucinations
- insomnia
- impotence
- loss of appetite

Behavioral and Social Symptoms of Addiction

- increased reliance on drugs
- family problems
- financial difficulties
- frequent change of jobs, lateness, other job-related problems
- car accidents
- increased legal problems from behavior
- suicidal behavior
- violent behavior
- suspiciousness
- unusually passive behavior

TEST YOURSELF FOR ADDICTION: FAIR OAKS SELF-TEST

Personal Drug-Use Inventory

This list of questions can help you decide whether you are misusing any chemicals, or have the potential for misusing them. There are no "good" or "bad" answers to many of them—only honest answers. But if you find yourself silently answering yes to more than a few, it may be time to start thinking about ways to reduce your use of drugs.

Are Drugs Affecting You Financially?

- Has spending money on drugs kept you from buying necessities, such as food or clothing, or from paying the rent or mortgage?
- Do you worry about how you'll pay for the drugs you use?
- Have you ever borrowed money to buy drugs?

Are Drugs Affecting Your Work?

- Have you ever missed a day's work because of using drugs?
- Have you ever used drugs for "fun" or to "help get through the day" while at work?

- Do your coworkers use drugs and try to get you to join them?
- Have you been worried lately about losing your job because of your use of drugs?

Do Drugs Get You Into Trouble?

- Have you ever driven a car while you've been under the influence of drugs and/or alcohol?
- Have you ever had an accident or been given a ticket while you were using drugs and/or alcohol?
- Have you lost a friend or friends because of your use of drugs?
- Do you lie about your drug use? Even to your close friends?
- Do you sometimes argue with people about the way you use drugs?

Do You Use Drugs for Nonmedical Reasons?

- Do you take drugs to improve your mood?
- Do you use drugs to improve your sexual performance?
- Do you take drugs to help you forget your problems?
- Do you sometimes take drugs before breakfast, perhaps to get the day off to a "good" start?

Do You Miss Drugs When You Stop Using Them?

- When you don't use drugs for a few days, do you feel depressed?
- Do you feel "left out" when you're not using drugs?
- Do you sometimes feel sick—a headache, upset stomach, etc.—when you stop taking drugs for a few days or a couple of weeks?

Does Your Use of Drugs Bother You at Times?

- Have you lost interest in sex—even a little—since you've been using drugs?
- Have you ever stopped taking drugs, even temporarily, because of an unpleasant physical or mental feeling?

- Have you ever felt sick while taking drugs but kept on taking them anyway?
- Have you ever tried to cut down your drug use?
- Do you sometimes worry that your drug use is out of control?
- Have you ever wondered whether you're addicted to drugs?
- Do you ever feel guilty about taking drugs?
- Do you have trouble waking up or feel like you have a hangover the morning after you use drugs?
- Do you suspect that your use of drugs has increased over the past few months?
- Do you think about drugs at least once a day? More often than that?

Are Drugs Affecting the Way You Think?

- Have you sometimes thought about suicide since you've been using drugs?
- Do you sometimes accept drugs without even asking what they are when a friend offers it to you?
- Are you sometimes unable to remember what happened after you've used drugs?
- Do you have trouble concentrating when you've taken drugs?[2]

2. The Fair Oaks Self-Test is taken from *The Little Black Pill Book*, Lawrence D. Chilnick, Editor in Chief. Copyright © 1983 by The Food and Drug Book Company, Inc. Reprinted by permission of Bantam Books, Inc. All rights reserved.

· 5 ·

People Enable Addiction —The Adolescent Story

How, you may ask, can someone let someone else—especially a child—reach the depths of addiction?

Most people don't realize they are. Many people unwittingly help those using drugs become addicts. They are the final component in the addiction equation, and we call them enablers. Here are some examples:

- A fifteen-year-old girl sees her brother smoking marijuana on the way home from school one day and doesn't tell her parents. Why not? She's afraid that he'll tell them about her sexual experimentation.
- A middle-class mother finds drug paraphernalia in her son's room and tells her husband. He ignores the problem and says with a sigh, "After all, we did it, it's only pot, and it's a phase they all go through."
- A teacher notes that a B-average student spends time nodding off in class and that her grades are dropping. At lunch the teacher notices that the student is hanging out with kids who are often absent and known to be drug users. The teacher does nothing because, after all, it's not her kid and she's only the history teacher, not a cop.
- A small-town police officer sees a sixteen-year-old boy exchanging drugs with another on the street. He simply turns his head

because last week he had confronted the kid's father at their club meeting. He's been politely told to mind his own business.

• A judge, knowing that jails are overcrowded and dangerous, sentences a second-time offender (for selling drugs) to a one-year probation and suspends the fine.

• A pediatrician treats a fifteen-year-old boy for a sinus problem and a cough with an antibiotic. He doesn't ask if he's using cocaine or crack and doesn't do a urine screen. He's worried that questioning the adolescent will "weaken the doctor/patient relationship."

• A psychotherapist sees a teenager for three months in therapy for behavioral problems. The patient admits that he uses drugs "on occasion." Yet the therapist continues to treat the patient without requiring drug screens and without making abstinence a part of their ground rules. After all, the therapist rationalizes, this might upset "the therapeutic alliance." The teen is often high at sessions, and the therapist either doesn't know or hopes to treat the drug problem by treating the "underlying" psychological problem.

With all of this emphasis on drugs, we forget an important part of the equation in the last chapter—people! These are examples of people who thought they were showing sensitivity and caring but were actually enabling the illness of addiction. People close to the drug user are just as much a part of the addictive process as the drug itself and the user's predisposition.

What does this mean to you as a parent or as a loved one of someone who's addicted? One of the most common questions asked of therapists by parents is, What did I do to cause this problem?

Parents of children in trouble with drugs feel guilt and embarrassment. Frequently this prevents them from seeking help sooner. As we look at all the factors that cause addiction—physiology, heredity, socioculture, and the drugs themselves—we feel very strongly that parents don't cause a kid to become addicted. We see many kids from good families who become addicted and many from terrible family situations who do not.

Since the gateway to teenage drug use in almost all cases is through peer groups, we try not to get parents and others involved with only the causes of addiction. Instead we try to focus on *what enables addiction*. What are they doing, we ask them, to allow the disease to progress to dependency and addiction?

The people in the examples didn't cause addiction, but they sure helped it along by their actions. Rarely is a single person in the addict's life responsible for this enabling. The teachers, brothers and sisters, the parents and the entire social structure all participated.

Enabling has a single common thread found throughout the addiction process—*denial*. Everyone in the drug user's world refuses to accept reality. Remember the stories in chapter three of the teenagers who spent thousands of dollars on drugs. How could their parents ignore what was going on in their basement? For many parents the answer is simply a need to protect themselves, their identity, or their position in the community from the threat of drug use by their children.

We have known about the extent of drug use for many years, if not the exact mechanism of addiction. *Denial is what has enabled the drug epidemic in this country.*

Denial is what has enabled the most frightening new trend in drug and alcohol use—the drop in age of the typical abuser. When the recreational drug era of the 1960s began, most abuse was confined to college age and older groups. But today adolescents are becoming more and more involved with all sorts of drugs, especially crack. Teenagers from diverse regions and economic classes are flooding treatment centers like Fair Oaks. Adolescence is difficult at best, and teenagers seem most prone to get involved with crack. Its power seems to "challenge them."

An even grimmer statistic is recent evidence that first use of drugs may be dropping *below* the junior high school level into the preteen age groups. Studies show that in the high school class of 1985, a significant proportion of drug users had tried drugs before tenth grade. About 60 percent of the marijuana users had their first experience with these drugs between the sixth and ninth grades.

Addiction is all too often fatal for young people. An astonishing fact is that fifteen-to-twenty-four-year-olds are the only age group with an increased death rate in the past ten years, mostly from drug-related accidents, suicides, and overdoses!

HOW TEENS USE DRUGS—
THE STAGES OF ABUSE

Teenagers today most frequently abuse alcohol, tobacco, marijuana, illegal prescription stimulants, and cocaine. Adolescents who smoke or drink are far more likely to abuse illegal drugs, and research has also shown that kids use more drugs in combination sooner than adults do.

Crack's low-cost "initiation fee" has made cocaine much more available and many times more dangerous to teens. So, ironically, the most vulnerable group—teenagers—is now most at risk for cocaine addiction. The social and personality factors we've seen in the teenagers in chapter three play directly into the hands of those selling low-cost, highly addictive drugs like crack. Teens who get into trouble with drugs go through several *stages* as they develop a full-blown addiction. If you recognize these stages or some of the signs and symptoms in the last part of chapter four, you may be able to act early enough to prevent a disaster.

Stage I: Experimentation

For many kids this stage begins in junior high school when, because of peer pressure, an adolescent decides to "try it." In general, this stage involves beer drinking, pot smoking, some inhalant sniffing. Usually the setting is at home, at a party, or wherever kids are just hanging out. Their motivation may be linked to the thrill that accompanies "acting grown-up" or defying parents' stated wishes.

Teens who first use drugs have a very low tolerance for the effects. The euphoria is usually followed by a quick return to normal, so no negative consequences or bad feelings accompany the experience. Drugs work on the pleasure centers in the brain, and for teens who are just beginning to experience a wide variety of sexual and other feelings, this sensation offers the seductive illusion that the drug is good for their bodies: What feels good must *be* good.

Stage II: Social-Recreational Use

Once the experimentation with drugs has begun, more regular use may develop, usually continuing with liquor or beer. Often they will use drugs or alcohol during the week, on school nights. And as more of the drug is being used, since tolerance is developing, they are often willing to suffer the consequences—hangovers and missed activities.

"Social-recreational" or "regular use" usually involves experimentation with a wide range of drugs from LSD to pills to crack. This in turn leads to a need for money to support the activity, which often leads to stealing money from home or dealing drugs.

Where do kids get drugs? Kids don't necessarily buy their drugs from the pusher in the schoolyard. That's another myth. Recent studies show that after initial introduction to a drug by a peer, 62 percent used income targeted for school lunches or expense money from part-time jobs to obtain cocaine. But then many turn to illegal activities to obtain money for drugs; 42 percent sold drugs. Both young men and women reported that they had used sexual means to obtain drugs.

One of the first signs parents may notice in this stage is a change in their teenager's social relationships. Nondrug-using friends are quickly dropped and a new group appears. Today we can go into many schools in the United States and readily identify two groups of teenagers: the straights and the druggies.

While in Stage I, teenagers learn how to go with the flow of the mood swings that accompany drug use. In Stage II, they actively seek that mood swing. Kids who begin to use drugs regularly know a lot about drugs—at least from their own viewpoint.

Some refer to themselves as junior chemists. They know exactly how much they need to get high and what effects it has on them after they use it. They also learn to hide the effects of their drug use from parents. Often, though, they may not be able to for long because this is the stage where the physical damage becomes obvious.

Drug abuse for teens is more dangerous than abuse among adults on almost every level, but especially physiologically. Teens who use drugs are far more vulnerable to developmental problems and even brain damage because their body's systems are not fully developed.

One main reason for health dangers to today's teens using drugs that must not be forgotten by parents who experimented with drugs in the 1960s is the potency difference between then and now. Today's drugs are many, many times more powerful than in the 1960s.

The marijuana is sometimes ten times more powerful. As we said in chapter one, "It's like the difference between a bicycle and a Sherman tank."

What about cocaine? Which drugs pose the greatest threat?

Cocaine abuse among teenagers is growing the fastest, partially fueled by the availability of crack. Recent studies show a leveling off of marijuana and alcohol use, but the spread of cocaine among teenagers continues. A recent study conducted by the Institute of Social Research at the University of Michigan shows that the number of high school seniors who have tried cocaine at least once has doubled in the past decade, from 9 percent to 17.3 percent.

Remember that all drug use is still widespread. Within the past year, almost half of all high school seniors, 49.6 percent, have used marijuana. Another 15.8 percent say they've used stimulants, and 13.8 percent used cocaine in the past year. Eighty percent of teenagers in one survey reported that marijuana was "easy to get."

Adolescents get into trouble with drugs and move through the process of addiction much faster than adults. A recent study conducted on our 800-COCAINE hot line of teen drug users showed that the time span from first use to a serious chronic problem was 15.5 months, compared to 4 to 4.5 years among adults. New data on crack use among teenagers show that they become addicted even sooner, perhaps in only a few months.

Overt symptoms of a drug problem may first appear in school. Our study showed that 75 percent of those using cocaine missed school more often than nonusers. Sixty-nine percent said their grades had dropped significantly, and 48 percent had suffered disciplinary problems. Thirty percent had been expelled from school.

How serious are the physical effects? Physical problems crop up almost immediately when kids abuse drugs. For example, 19 percent reported seizure that led to unconsciousness, 13 percent had auto accidents, 14 percent had tried suicide, and an astounding 27 percent reported violent behavior on drugs. Sinus problems, rhinitis, headaches, nausea, vomiting, poor appetite, and weight loss are chronic physical complaints of teenage cocaine users.

Emotional problems accompany each of the different stages of drug abuse and appear very quickly once regular use begins. For example, jitteriness, anxiety, depression, insomnia, and fatigue were reported by more than two-thirds of those surveyed. Others

said they suffered from delusions, paranoia, and compulsive behavior. Almost two-thirds of the teenagers using drugs said they had
lost their ability to concentrate and had memory loss.

Some of these problems are specific to cocaine, but teenagers
using only marijuana reported similar behavioral, social, and academic problems. They have also cited difficulties when stopping
use, reporting that they've felt irritable, nauseous, and suffered
insomnia, and many mentioned traffic accidents, since marijuana
use impairs coordination and driving skills.

One other serious effect occurs when teenagers use drugs regularly: the *amotivational syndrome*. It is one of the most significant
signs that drug use—especially marijuana use—has progressed to a
serious level. Kids experience fatigue, loss of interest in any activity,
and very low motivation. Because drug use leads to many other
problems—for example, being dropped from a team or school play,
sinking grades, or even lying to parents and friends—they also
suffer emotional pain and guilt.

This phase will often include a significant event—a fight at home,
failure on an important exam, or a break up with a boyfriend or girlfriend. At this point the teenager recalls only that "drugs make me
feel good" or "help me forget." The drug is substituted for coping,
and drug use becomes more than an occasional occurrence. A strong
sense of denial begins as teenagers cannot accept that there is any
association between their drug use and the consequences of what is
happening in their lives.

Stage III: Preoccupation

When drug use becomes *more* than a regular event, a teenager will
often become involved with even more damaging drugs—heroin,
crack, speed, PCP, and others. By this stage many kids are suffering
the symptoms listed above.

Teenagers who reach this stage may or may not still be going to
school. If they are in school, they often just sit there, preoccupied
with thinking about drugs. They spend their time planning their
next drug buy, thinking, Who will I buy what drugs from; who will I
get high with tonight? Thoughts of drugs replace thoughts of family,
school, or friends. Being high is the major preoccupation, and they
are high most of the time. Because they need more money, theft

becomes acceptable, along with lying and cheating. As a result of their compulsion, they may have run-ins with the police and other officials.

Some teenagers at this stage recognize the consequences and try to stop. Usually they are unable to, and feel guilt and shame as they realize that their drug use is out of control and there's nothing they can do about it. They take more and more drugs to self-medicate. It's a vicious cycle of use, fighting the cravings for more as the drug wears off and then getting high again. The harm to themselves and others worsens.

Stage IV: Dependency

Finally, they are addicted. And often they are addicted to everything. They are injecting, smoking crack, using drugs before school, during school, after school—totally out of control. They don't even know what normal is anymore.

Self-image, very important to teens, is connected only with drugs. With the increase of guilt, their self-image becomes lower, and their self-hatred leads to thoughts about suicide. In our 800-COCAINE surveys, we found that fully 18 percent of adolescents using cocaine had attempted suicide, and 36 percent had thought about it.

By this time, as we saw in the case of Linda, most adults recognize that they need help, but not most teenagers. They are mired in their despair, feelings of guilt, and negative self-image. Many can't get treatment on their own or are so far gone that no one wants to help them. All too often the resolution of this problem is the death of an otherwise fine young person whose body has been taken over by the drug.

Can Denial Be Defeated?

Another reason denial develops is a concept known as *codependency*. This refers to an emotional dependency that one person may have on an addict. As humans, we value our ability to enter into emotional relationships. It's a primary urge found in infants and carried out into adulthood. Some studies even suggest that infants need these emotional relationships to survive physically. Naturally, parents are attached to teenagers. When the teenager begins to use drugs, this emotional attachment often becomes codependency.

The parent can actually become dependent on the teenager in a way that is similar to the addict's dependency on his drugs. The codependent person will have his mood altered by the addict in a way that is similar to the way the addict's behavior and emotional state is altered by the drug. It's often this close emotional attachment that occurs among addicts and parents or teachers or other close friends that leads them to deny someone's drug use around them.

A Common Story

We had one case of a boss whose first employee was very instrumental in helping the company get off the ground. Over the years the boss helped his assistant through her divorce and a nasty child-custody suit. When the assistant became involved with someone who obviously used drugs, the boss chose to ignore the problem. He was dependent, he thought, on that person for his effectiveness. When the assistant became drug-impaired, he also ignored all of the signs, stages, and warnings. Soon it was too late. When the assistant's behavior became clearly harmful to the business, she was fired.

Interestingly, the boss never confronted her and never offered her help. To this day, the boss has never been able to see his old friend and associate after learning that drugs were the cause of her behavior.

It's often this close emotional attachment that allows people to ignore the reality of the drug abuse of their children or fellow workers. Parents have told us how they have been nervous or cautious or protective around their households for months before "the crisis." They had no idea how this was related to the drug-using behavior of their teenager. Only in the end, when a kid was picked up by the police or suffered a near-fatal overdose, were they aware of how closely linked their behavior was to that of their child.

There are two other aspects of denial that we will talk more about in a later chapter. One is the drug use of the enablers or parents themselves. The other is a lack of accurate knowledge about drugs. We will cover this more fully in our plan for a solution to the drug problem. Both of these contribute to the process of denial. But for now let us focus on a major part of denial—lack of knowledge of what to look for.

WHAT ARE THE MOST IMPORTANT SIGNALS?

While there is disagreement among experts about the importance of personality traits as a predictor of drug use, there is some agreement about common behavior among teens in trouble with drugs. Most feel adolescents who use and abuse alcohol, marijuana, and other illegal drugs almost always have one or more of the following in common:

- Peer drug use and approval
- A feeling that drug use is acceptable and essentially harmless
- Nonconforming, rebellious behavior
- Lowered grades in school
- Parental drug use or approval
- Behavior that most adults do not accept as normal for teens, including use of cigarettes, delinquent acts

Just as adult users display some physical and behavioral signs and symptoms, adolescents have similar "warning signals" that may mean they're in trouble and their drug experimentation has gotten out of hand. Although the following is not a diagnosis, these are common traits among adolescents today. Some fit in with the list above, too.

Behavioral Signs of Drug Abuse

- Chronic lying about whereabouts
- Sudden disappearance of money or valuables from home
- Marked dysphoric mood changes that occur without good reason and that cause pain to the family or patient

- Abusive behavior toward self or others
- Frequent outbursts of poorly controlled hostility with lack of insight or remorse for this behavior

Social Signs of Drug Abuse

- Driving while impaired, auto accidents
- Frequent truancy
- Underachievement over past six to twelve months with definite deterioration of academic performance

Circumstantial Evidence of Drug Abuse

- Drugs or drug paraphernalia in room, clothes, or car
- Drug terminology in school notebooks or in school yearbook
- Definitive change in peer-group preference to those who are already associated with drug use

Physical Symptoms of Drug Abuse

- Chronic fatigue or lethargy
- Chronic dry, irritating cough; chronic sore throat
- Chronic conjunctivitis (red eyes) otherwise unexplained

WHAT CAN YOU DO?

Once a teenager's parents have broken through their wall of denial, they often don't know what to do first.

There are as many answers as there are points along the chemical dependency road at which to intervene. But one thing is necessary—a *confrontation*. By this we don't mean yelling and screaming or fighting and threatening someone. Instead the drug user must be confronted with his or her behavior and consequences of the drug user's behavior must be pointed out to him. Their wall of denial must be breached, too.

How do you do this?

It must be done with an attitude of *caring*, and not in an angry tone. But above all it must be done honestly. If the drug user's activity makes one feel embarrassed, then this should be said: "I feel embarrassed when I have to tell my friends that you have quit the sports team and that your grades have dropped, but I'm more worried that you were picked up by the police for drinking and driving. You could hurt yourself!"

But a confrontation isn't easy. Many parents say, "I can't get them to listen," or, "They simply run away from me when I try to talk to them."

All of the above may and probably will happen. Many kids know how to manipulate parents and perhaps frighten them into backing down. If that happens, the process of addiction will simply continue. That is why it's important to *hold your ground*. Define what is acceptable behavior and what is not.

This is an important first step in breaking the cycle of drug addiction. These actions can often lead to what is really needed—getting the person into treatment.

·6·
Getting the Right Treatment

Perhaps the reason why stories told by people in treatment are so horrendous is that it is firsthand testimony from those who have let their drug problems progress far beyond the crisis level. Most people build a wall of denial around their drug addiction. Their friends and loved ones often deny the problem too. Frequently the wall must collapse totally before someone will accept treatment. Then too often it's too late to avoid hospitalization or other long-term treatment, and much suffering and damage has already occurred.

A drug abuser, like a person trying to quit smoking or gambling, may make several attempts at self-limiting. "I'll stop on Monday after one more binge," is a common refrain. But finally a severe financial, marital, or job-related crisis they can't handle appears. Like Linda in chapter four, faced with loss of their jobs and with only suicide or death as an option, they finally seek help. Interestingly, our studies show that cocaine abusers are willing to give up almost any aspect of their lives *but* their jobs before they will admit they need help. The job is usually their link to the drugs. It provides the money or the dealer. Cocaine is unique in this respect. Others who abuse opiates like heroin or even marijuana users often give up work *first* because they can't work while using those drugs. Cocaine users, in the early stages of the addictive process, can continue to work.

It's vital to assess a person's motivation and sincerity when he seeks treatment. Frequently a person seeking treatment will do so only to appease those around him. If the drug user can manipulate those who are his enablers then, he hopes, he will not have to give up drugs altogether. By appeasing those who seek to help them, drug users may only be seeking an "easy out" like a treatment program that does not demand enforced abstinence.

TREATMENT MYTHS

Why do people who know they are in trouble with drugs—or at the very least using "too much"—wait until their lives crumble before they accept help? What is the reason that so many people resist treatment for drug abuse? We know that denial is a common trait among anyone chemically dependent, but that's not the only reason someone may resist an offer of help. As in all aspects of drug abuse, treatment has spawned its own myths that can block a helping hand.

Many people, for example, think that getting off drugs always involves "going cold turkey." Abrupt withdrawal, followed by days of nightmarish sweating, nausea, vomiting, and other horrors of detoxification are all part of the price many think you have to pay for stopping being a "junkie."

This myth is often accompanied by another seemingly less dangerous one: Once you get off drugs, you're cured. After all, it's just a matter of willpower to break your old habits and associations with the other users who dragged you into the abyss.

Many people who used drugs casually in the 1960s still believe these myths, which contribute to the reluctance on the part of many to get treatment early, rather than at the crisis stage of an addiction. Users rationalize, "Why do something now? I have a little fun with drugs now and then stop whenever I want." Teenagers often think, "I'll stop when I'm twenty."

Some people, especially parents, have become fearful and cautious about treatment programs. Because of recent attention to the drug problem, media coverage has exposed some abuses in the treatment field. Many of these focus on the lack of adequate supervision, especially by a physician, and on the staff confronting patients. Since drug addiction has many medical and psychiatric consequences, it is always important to have a qualified physician (usually a psychiatrist) to supervise treatment. This person should be available initially to attend to any symptoms of withdrawal as well as to assess the need for additional medical or psychiatric treatment. Some addicts may need treatment such as antidepressant medication. Some family members and professionals are reluctant to treat the addicts with such medications as antidepressants or lithium (for manic-depressive illness) for fear that they are addicting. These drugs are not addicting. They work by restoring a biochemical balance to normal so that a person can function better. This is often a necessary ingredient of treatment.

The role and manner of confrontation in treatment has often been misunderstood. Addicts have developed a strong wall of denial and personal defenses about their drug use and behavior. To overcome the denial and defenses, confrontation is usually necessary. But a successful treatment program should not interpret confrontation as beating, yelling, or humiliating the person, but as pointing out to the person certain manifestations and consequences of their actions. For instance, saying, "I feel intimidated when you are silent and stare at me with your jaw clenched. I get afraid that you will hit me rather than talk to me." Often, because of denial, addicts are unaware of their own actions or the effect that they have on others. This behavior must be changed to achieve a successful recovery, since much of it is a result of, may be associated with, or lead to, future drug use if not changed.

But the myths about treatment don't end here.

Another treatment myth involves the type of drug a person uses. Many people feel that if they beat an addiction to one drug, they can safely use another without risking addiction again. Nothing could be further from the truth.

Crack is the perfect example. Someone who recovers from an addiction to crack, pills, or even marijuana is a sitting duck for the lure of alcohol. Alcohol use can quickly lead to its own addiction or it may lower restraints enough to have the user return to "trying" crack. Addiction, remember, is a complex process involving loss of control, and compulsive and repeated use without regard to the consequences. The pattern of use will be the same, no matter what drug is involved. In addition, the chance of a person formerly addicted to any other drug using crack only a single time without using it again borders on zero.

WHAT IS THE REALITY?

Today addiction treatment is much more sophisticated than "cold turkey in a padded cell." It often involves using a variety of drugs to mitigate the effects of withdrawal to help someone through the cravings that they feel after detoxification. Modern treatment programs involve many different techniques and are tailored to the patient, depending on age, health status, type of drug use, and other factors.

In fact, for many people treatment may be the most exciting and best event that happened in their lives. The recovery process is structured to reveal insights about themselves and assist in developing self-esteem and learning new coping skills. It's usually experienced as being given a "second chance" in life. I know one cocaine-addicted physician who states, "It gave me back my life!" It is also wonderful and heartwarming to hear parents at our graduation from treatment say, "It is hard for me to express how grateful I am to the program for having given back my family!" Much has been changed, and this is the beginning in the road to recovery.

CAN YOU CURE YOURSELF?

Many people believe that once you have gotten a drug out of your system or you aren't using drugs compulsively—without control and regard to the consequences—you are safe.

A person who is addicted is never cured. He may be "sober" or "drug-free," but once you suffer from addictive disease, you will always have the potential to relapse into the same sort of drug-using behavior as before. Often in a relapse the dependency develops more rapidly and more severely than previously. Initially, each day is a struggle for recovering addicts. That's why most people who are recovering tell you they have learned to take life "one day at a time." Recovering from addiction is a lifelong process.

HOW DO YOU KNOW YOU NEED TREATMENT?

Half the battle to beating drug abuse involves getting help early, and the other half is knowing what kind of help to seek. Inpatient hospitalization and a comprehensive outpatient program are the options. Therefore the key to getting help for any type of drug problem is finding the right treatment program. (Note: If you have no access to any drug program in your area, you can call 800-CO-CAINE, the twenty-four-hour national helpline, to get further information about treatment and a personal referral.)

In general, an outpatient treatment program is preferable to hospitalization because it can be used by almost anyone who has no serious health-related problems (i.e., blood infections from needles, cardiac or central-nervous-system damage) or needs to detoxify immediately. It's also more acceptable to many people from a social standpoint. However, with the levels of substance abuse found in many workplaces today, entering treatment carries less of a stigma. Also, recent studies done by 800-COCAINE show that eight out of ten employers would rather get an employee treatment than fire him for drug abuse. The cost today to replace even an unskilled laborer is between five and seven thousand dollars.

1. How severe is the drug abuse problem?
   - Is his drug use so uncontrollable that he can't stop at all?
   - Is he using large doses of drugs? Is he using dangerous methods such as freebasing, injecting, or smoking?
   - Is he using several drugs?
2. How severe are his behavioral and emotional problems?
   - Is the user's daily function interrupted?
   - Can he take care of himself, go to work, relate to other people?
   - Is he so paranoid or so depressed that he cannot think clearly?
   - Has the person become suicidal or violent?
3. Have other medical problems occurred such as sinus, heart, liver, or systemic infections?
4. Has the patient failed in other outpatient attempts?

These questions should help you see a clearer pattern in the person's drug use.

If there are few yesses and a treatment specialist agrees, outpatient treatment is the treatment of choice for most drug abusers, especially cocaine powder users not yet using crack since many can usually stop quickly without substitute drugs for withdrawal.

In general people who fit the outpatient profile are in the early stages of drug abuse. They do not have a full blown addiction and are highly motivated to stop. They are probably willing to agree to give up all drugs and enter an outpatient program that includes many of the aspects we'll talk about later in this chapter. The main characteristics of a successful outpatient are that he be willing to participate in a program that has urine screening to ensure abstinence and to attend frequent meetings and support groups. Most programs will require at the start that the outpatient sign a "contract" for eight to ten weeks. At the end of that period there will be a reevaluation.

Outpatient treatment is usually much less expensive and is less disruptive and stigmatizing to the patient's overall lifestyle and job.

If the person is not out of control and is strongly motivated to be drug free, then with family support he or she may be expected to succeed. People who functioned well before they got into trouble with drugs can usually function well after drug cessation. If they can make the lifestyle changes needed and incorporate total abstinence into their lives, there is a high probability of success no matter which type of treatment is used.

In general the more "yesses," the more likely it is that hospitalization will be needed. Unfortunately, hospitalization sometimes can't be avoided. Some people's drug abuse may be so out of control that their lives are in danger from a secondary disease or a severe depression brought on by drug use.

The indications for hospitalization will include a combination of:

- Compulsive IV use or freebase use
- Concurrent physical dependency presenting clear psychiatric and physical problems
- Severe impairment of social or family functioning
- A strong resistance to treatment or failure in other outpatient treatment attempts.

Once you have a handle on the severity of the problem, you can make a decision about the kind of treatment to seek.

The first thing you should ask about a drug treatment program is How successful is it? It's a natural question—and a fair one, but not that simple to answer, since the success rates of any type of program depend on the person as much as the program.

HOW TO CHOOSE A PROGRAM

Before you decide where to go, you should consider several aspects of any program. Visit with every staff person with whom you or your loved one will come in contact. Check the references and the history of the program carefully. Financial questions such as insurance coverage, length of stay that will be covered, and any hidden costs are very important. Seeking drug treatment is certainly as important a medical decision as seeking a doctor to perform surgery. Certainly you would not let an inexperienced surgeon perform a bypass on you just to save a few dollars or because the surgeon needed experience. Like most aspects of medical choice, word of mouth can often help you find a good place to start looking.

But seeking treatment for drug abuse is not the same as looking for a surgeon for heart disease since many people feel there is a stigma attached to drug problems. So if you can't ask a friend or someone close to you, like a member of the clergy or a teacher, examine a program in the following manner as suggested by Dr. Mark S. Gold in *The Facts About Drugs and Alcohol:*[1]

1. Does the program require total, immediate abstinence from all drug use? Any occasional drug use during treatment is unrealistic and dangerous to the person in treatment. Anyone who uses drugs while seeking help is not really going to succeed. Any program you choose *must* insist on complete abstinence.

2. Does the program require urine testing? This is a critical and indispensable aspect of any outpatient program. A sample must be taken one to two times per week. This builds mutual trust between the patient and the clinician. When there is no

1. Used by permission.

question that the addict is not using, there is no need for the patient to build the denial and self-deceit that is so common to drug abusers. Urine testing helps promote self-control over drug urges. The program should make clear at the outset the consequences for any "slipping" that does occur. These could include temporary suspension from the program, more intensive, individualized contact, or even mandatory hospitalization.

Urine testing in the workplace is a very controversial topic and is in fact the subject of another entire book. But urine testing as part of treatment for drug addiction is not, in our minds, an issue of controversy. There is absolutely no way at all to shake an addiction if you continue to use drugs. Testing urine is the only accurate way to determine if someone has been using drugs. When we test for drugs in treatment, we are seeking the presence of drugs, not the level of impairment, as one would in the workplace. While drug testing is a matter of court battles in some venues, it's not a matter of controversy for drug-treatment programs that work. You can go to many outpatient programs that don't require urine testing and be told, "We can spot a drug user by behavior." Don't allow someone you love to go into that program. He will never be drug-free. A program that demands abstinence and then enforces it through testing is a must.

3. Does the program have a clear-cut "road to recovery" program? A good outpatient program should have three "phases" that can overlap.

Phase I is *Initial abstinence*, which may last from thirty to sixty days with the emphasis on getting someone totally drug-free for at least one month. This time period is suggested because it seems realistic to most people and within their capability. During this phase people are seen almost every day by a trained professional. They receive counseling, support, and education. During this time the concept of denial is discussed, and patients seek answers to the reasons they have resisted giving up drugs. After two to three weeks, the patient is brought into a recovery group of his peers.

Powerful urges and cravings for drugs can develop in this phase, so the counselors try to identify the "stimuli" that cause these urges for the patient. Unless the patient is properly warned about the process, the urges come out of nowhere, it seems. These cravings, which may be the result of depletion of neurotransmitters in the brain or learned associations, can overpower the patient, and he will be unable to avoid returning to the drugs.

Some patients feel that once a craving begins it can't be resisted. This is yet another myth. These cravings are always temporary, and the patient should learn behavior modification methods to repel them. For example, change environment or avoid seeing other people who trigger memories of past drug use. Other quick-action methods, such as seeking out family or friends who will nullify these feelings, are also used.

In addition, certain drugs like bromocriptine help reduce cravings and drug urges among cocaine users. This drug, which is usually used as a treatment for Parkinson's disease, seems to mask the withdrawal symptoms caused by dopamine depletion when cocaine is used. (See page 18.) Often cravings or drug urges occur when another feeling is being avoided. In treatment we usually see drug urges occurring when a person is afraid or lonely. By recognizing this underlying feeling, a person can act in a healthy way to relieve the feeling rather than using drugs to avoid it.

Phase II includes *relapse prevention* and lifestyle-change directions. The patient should learn the most common and predictable factors that lead to drug relapse and should help alter his lifestyle comfortably to avoid future drug use. Patients also learn to recognize and avoid early warning signs and "setups," or times when they unconsciously put themselves into a situation in which they will be open to drug use.

Patients should also be counseled about Abstinence Violation Effect (AVE), which is very common among those attempting to shake drug addiction. AVE refers to the predictable defeatist reaction that is commonly experienced by an abstaining user after he's had a slip. The slip will set off a complex set of intense negative feelings of failure, guilt, and self-loathing for having "given in." Family members and patients should be prepared to accept a slip and learn how to combat an AVE. Part of the process of recovery, especially with teenagers, is relapse. The destructive consequences of the AVE should be recognized and not be allowed to nullify or derail the recovery process.

Phase III is *consolidation,* which begins after the first year of treatment and lasts indefinitely. This may include participation in "senior" group therapy and the learning of other tasks, such as how to avoid "flare-up periods," combatting overconfidence and other psychological problems that were suppressed by drug use.

4. What about self-help group programs? Joining a group program is an invaluable component of any outpatient treatment. Some self-help programs like Alcoholics Anonymous, Cocaine Anonymous, and others are very effective. In fact, over one million people each day attend AA meetings. But self-help groups must be supervised by qualified people. Ideally, a group should meet and be led by a recovering person who has been abstinent for several years. This group should be part of a comprehensive program that includes individual, family, or other modes of therapy.

There are a lot of advantages to a self-help group. But therapeutic adjunct groups must be part of a drug-free environment in which urine tests are given to participants.

One advantage to a group is that different patients will be in different stages of recovery, which helps the newer members gain the benefit of role models. Living examples are the best tools for recovery. Groups also promote rapid learning and educational experience on a wide variety of personalized recovery issues. The groups can also focus on specific techniques that work in the "real world." These also help overcome shame and guilt associated with drug use. Plus, the group's attitude can be an important method for maintaining motivation to stay drug-free.

Many people resist the idea of a group at first because of privacy issues or the discomfort involved in sharing personal problems with strangers. But adjustment is usually very rapid, and after the first few sessions most people respond well.

And, as mentioned, recovery groups keep the process moving forward after a long period of abstention.

6. What is the family's role?

Close family members, especially a spouse or parents, should be involved in any drug-treatment program. As mentioned previously, well-intentioned family members often function as enablers by making excuses for the abuser or providing money to spare the abuser from suffering the consequences of this negative behavior. Family members must learn their roles in helping the person remain drug-free, as we mentioned in chapter five. The program must instruct the family how to deal with a recovering addict through all the phases of treatment. Family members should get support and education by joining the self-help groups of Families Anonymous or Alanon to deal with issues of co-dependency. (See Referrals at the back of the book.)

7. Are there any other aspects to treatment? Often an inpatient drug-treatment program requires detoxification with use of other medication—like naltrexone or clonidine. Clonidine, brand name Catapres, has been shown to be the first nonaddictive, nonnarcotic treatment for opiate withdrawal. Clonidine fools the brain into thinking it's not in withdrawal when it is. Using clonidine, a person addicted to heroin or methadone can be drug-free in ten to fourteen days. Naltrexone blocks the opiate receptors in the brain, which are literally the landing sites for heroin. Thus the heroin has no effect at all. If you inject heroin while using naltrexone, it will simply be excreted. If administered properly it can make the user relapse- and overdose-"proof."

Some programs offer regularly scheduled exercise and relaxation programs that can be an important part of recovery. Other programs deal with stress reduction or workaholism that can be part of an overall lifestyle pattern that leads to drug abuse.

Addiction treatment can work and be a very beneficial step. Unfortunately, people often resist the "drastic" step, even when it's obviously required. Never forget, it is better to have a living addict who's been hospitalized and properly withdrawn than an addict whose life has been lost because he or his family didn't want him committed. The most important aspect of treatment is that it happen. Getting someone help often falls on the shoulders of a family member or a loved one when users can't help themselves. Don't be afraid to lose "friendship" temporarily. You might lose a loved one permanently if you fail to act.

The answer is finding a program that follows the above concepts and matches the criteria we've described. If you cannot find a program that meets these specifications, contact 800-COCAINE directly, and they will help you find the right treatment program.

Remember, treatment may be the most important and exciting event in a drug addict's life!

•7•
Crack and Crime— The True Story

According to the Drug Enforcement Administration (DEA) officials, crack is one of the most interesting and clearly the most *frightening* crime story to appear in many years.

"A little over one year ago, I heard my first mention of crack," Robert M. Stutman, Special Agent in charge of the New York office of the DEA, told us. "That was in May 1985, and it was a single mention in a two-hour meeting. We didn't even make our first sizable seizure until months later, in October 1985."

Today Agent Stutman, a twenty-two-year veteran in the DEA, says it is now the single biggest drug threat his federal agency has to deal with. Crack and cocaine have recently supplanted heroin, which had been the DEA's number-one priority for twenty years.

"I thought when I first heard about it that it was a fad," Stutman says. "But less than a year later, one of every three drug arrests in rural Georgia—not to mention New York—involves crack! I find that amazing."

The cocaine trade, which spawned the crack business, *is* amazing. It certainly has had a long history, since cocaine has been with us for quite some time. Here are some of the highlights of the history of cocaine.[1]

---

1. From *The Facts About Drugs and Alcohol* by Dr. Mark S. Gold, copyright © 1986 by Fair Oaks Hospital. Used by permission.

The coca plant—*Erythroxylon coca*—is indigenous to the eastern Andes mountains of South America. The plant is thought to predate the appearance of man. Cocaine is only one of the fourteen alkaloids in its leaves. The bitter taste and anesthetic qualities probably evolved as chemical defenses to ward off animals anticipating a good meal of fresh greenery. Coca today remains relatively free of insect pests, and grazing animals seldom bother the plants. With careful tending, coca has been grown in Southeast Asia, central Europe, and the United States, but never in large enough quantities to become a major source of cocaine. Contrary to common myths, and despite the similar-sounding name, the plant is related to neither the stubby tree providing chocolate (*Theobroma cacao*) nor the coconut palm (*Cocos nucifera*).

Of the 250 varieties of coca, only two possess enough cocaine to make them economically interesting to farmers. These are planted in hillside rows where rainfall is abundant and temperatures moderate, and are kept well-trimmed to make harvesting as easy as possible. Other plants generating substantial international trade—corn and wheat, for example—have been genetically altered to develop improved strains. Coca plants cultivated today are almost identical to coca plants grown millions of years ago. Coca plants have always been an important cash crop. Coca bushes, in fact, may be the most valuable naturally occurring plants in the world.

As much as 77 million pounds of dried coca leaves are grown each year in Bolivia alone. That's three times more than the country produced a mere decade ago. And Bolivia is not the world's sole source of cocaine: Peru grows 66 million pounds annually.

Historically, the Incas used the coca plant sacramentally in religious rituals. The leaves were a good-luck charm to attract love and wealth, and were part of initiation rites, weddings, and even burial ceremonies. By 1750, specimens had reached European researchers, who classified the plant according to scientific standards, but not until the late eighteenth century did detailed reports of the plant's virtues begin to spread in Europe.

In 1855, the powerful cocaine alkaloid was isolated from the raw leaf. Almost immediately cocaine became popular among Europeans both as a medicine and a pleasure drug. A few years later, Corsican chemist Angelo Mariani introduced the public to the first coca-containing elixir, "Vin Mariani." With a reputation as a cure-all, it was endorsed by everyone from Thomas Edison to Pope Leo XIII. With an entrepreneurial spirit almost unheard of a century ago, the chemist came even closer than Timothy Leary to "turning on" the world.

In 1886 a health drink called Coca-Cola came on the scene. It was the predecessor of today's popular soft drink and "the first generally advertised product that directed people to a drug store," according to researcher-author Robert Wilson. The beverage was served at soda fountains across the country, and its nickname, Coke, became the popular name of the drink's active ingredient, cocaine.

Within a few years there were dozens of similar beverages on the market, all containing cocaine. Men, women, and children alike visited drug stores for a "pick-me-up" of soda laced with cocaine. It was not until the purer form of the drug became available in medical practice that the real dangers surfaced.

Throughout the 1880s, medical enthusiasm for cocaine rose steadily. Sigmund Freud's landmark 1884 paper, "On Coca," described the drug's effects on himself and outlined a half dozen major uses for cocaine: as a stimulant; for digestive disorders; to cure morphine addiction; to treat asthma; as an aphrodisiac; and as a local anesthetic. Only the last of these proved to be valid at all. The founder of psychoanalysis was more interested in cocaine's medicinal potential than its potential adverse effects. Used in moderation, he concluded, cocaine was "more likely to promote health than impair it."

Firmly convinced of cocaine's benefits, Freud treated the morphine habit of a physician friend Ernst von Fleischl-Marxow by substituting cocaine for the supposedly more dangerous morphine. But the doctor's cocaine use got out of hand, and he began to suffer from toxic symptoms.

This combination of cocaine with an opiate like heroin or morphine, later used by modern drug addicts, became known as "the speedball" and was responsible for the recent death of actor John Belushi.

Credit for using cocaine as an anesthetic deservedly goes to Carl Koller, an associate of Freud's at Vienna General Hospital, who supported its use for ophthalmic procedures. Until then, eye operations had been performed without anesthesia; they were extremely painful and difficult to accomplish.

Because the drug rapidly became a favorite for "repeat users" in 1901, the American Pharmacological Association set up the Committee on the Acquirement of the Drug Habit, which condemned cocaine and its manufacturers with equal vehemence.

The Pure Food and Drug Act of 1906 severely restricted the use of cocaine in patent medicines and tonics. It had already been eliminated from Coca-Cola and many similar elixirs, being replaced by various flavoring agents and less controversial drugs like caffeine. But as late as 1909, nearly seventy Coca-Cola imitations—with cocaine—remained on the market. (Coca-Cola now uses South American coca leaves treated to remove all traces of cocaine.)

In the early 1900s cocaine's use for all but medicinal purposes was, at long last, outlawed. The Harrison Narcotics Act made cocaine illegal but misclassified it as a narcotic. A labyrinth of federal and state laws restricting cocaine forced the drug far underground but did not eliminate its illegal use.

Although cocaine was buried, it was still alive. Though public interest in cocaine waned from the twenties through the early sixties, the drug remained popular among society's mavericks, mainly well-connected entertainers and the less respectable wealthy. It came to symbolize chic, high-society decadence. Among the poor, its price made cocaine an almost unobtainable drug, although some users managed to find affordable sources by dealing it.

The 1960s introduced a new attitude toward illicit drugs among the large middle-class population just coming of age. Drug abuse was only one facet of the widespread changes our society experienced, but it was one that would alter the focus and tenor of the way coke was used.

Cocaine next became widely available in this country during the late 1960s, more because of supply than demand. As a result it is without any doubt one of the most profitable industries known to capitalists anywhere. To some extent, its latest renaissance is a classic entrepreneurial rags-to-riches story. In fact, no less an authoritative source than *The Wall Street Journal* has reported its growth.

On June 30, 1986, the *Journal* called the cocaine industry, "Latin America's only successful multinational," and reported on it in this sober fashion:

Ten years ago, for instance, the cocaine trade was a haphazard cottage industry. Since then it has moved away from its entrepreneurial origins and through a brutal shakeout. Now, relatively stable and dominated by a few well-entrenched giants, it increasingly looks like a maturing industry. It has saturated its prime market, the U.S., and probably has seen its profit margins narrow. Over the next few years, it may even see the U.S. market begin to shrink.

The *Journal,* also reported: "In response to these changes, it is looking to new products, such as crack—a potent form of cocaine that is smoked—and to new markets such as Europe. Meanwhile, as the industry grows to value discretion, Los Angeles may be replacing Miami as its U.S. headquarters." While *The Wall Street Journal* may see the cocaine story as a business success, only coincidence has led to its current multibillion-dollar status. Here's why cocaine today is reaching pandemic proportions.

Until the late sixties few people knew about or wanted cocaine. It was a relatively limited cash crop in Colombia where more exotic strains of marijuana were the major source of income. In the mid 1970s, most U.S. pot came from Mexico until the U.S. government convinced the Mexican government to eradicate its marijuana crop. About the same time, many South American and Cuban refugees found themselves with plenty of spare time on their fishing boats because they were excluded by regional laws from lobstering near the Bahamas.

Supply met demand in a classic new business venture, and Colombian marijuana began to flood the U.S. market via the idle boats in the Caribbean and off the Florida coast. At the same time, we also saw the growth of the U.S. marijuana industry, which today amounts to an annual crop of over 2000 tons, 25 percent of which is sinsemilla, a strain of marijuana ten times more powerful than the marijuana of the 1960s imported from Mexico.

Once the Colombians had established a distribution system in the mid- to late 1970s, the cocaine era was on. Marijuana, they quickly discovered, was bulky and risky to import. So they switched to cocaine, which is compact, lighter, and easier to conceal. Through clever "marketing" techniques and because the drug was used by those who were rich and famous and could afford it, coke caught on again.

According to the DEA, in 1976 about 19 metric tons of cocaine were imported. By 1982, that amount had risen to 45 metric tons.

The rest of the cocaine story has been pretty well documented in the popular press, which has followed the story as closely as the *Journal* and other national media. Virtually every national publication and major TV network has covered the drug story in the past few years. Programs like the fall 1986 CBS News documentary "48 Hours on Crack Street" revealed the severity of the problem and uncovered some of the horrors associated with it. In this show, Dan Rather investigated a vermin-infested crack house, and cameras focused on black teenagers in New York City's Times Square smoking crack. As one of the people who treats crack addicts, especially kids, I worry that the glamour and sensationalism obscure the fact that the epidemic isn't limited to New York or to blacks. In fact, my fear is that programs like the CBS documentary will convince people in suburbia and outside urban ghettos that they are safe.

Nothing could be further from the truth. Crack has changed the nature of the cocaine business once again. Before crack appeared, the price of cocaine was declining in the U.S. as supplies grew. From 1982 to 1985, the price of a gram—the typical amount purchased by a regular user—dropped from $125 to $75. One reason was that domestic labs were being set up to break down the coca paste into base. These labs were safer and cheaper to set up here than south of the border where ether, a needed ingredient in the process, is twenty times more expensive.

In chapter two we said that crack is only different from cocaine in its form and route of use. Well, it actually is different in one other important respect, according to DEA agent Stutman. "Crack," he says, "really is a cottage industry today. Although it may not be that way a year from now, today crack does not come from any single source or a single controlling group. This is exactly the opposite of the cocaine hydrochloride business."

Since crack can be made by anyone with baking soda in an eight-minute process, it has mushroomed into a growing business for any entrepreneur with access to the tiny vials and the cocaine HCL that is easily purchased from the already established cocaine industry.

Crack dealers don't need a central source of supply, so anyone can go into this very profitable business with little overhead and relative safety. The trafficking patterns of crack, according to the DEA, are not parallel to those of the cocaine HCL business, which is run by a very tight, organized system. Today, crack labs and dealers can spring up anywhere. And no one, the DEA admits, knows why—at least yet.

"We don't know why there's so much crack in rural Georgia, but very little in Atlanta, for example," says Mr. Stutman.

We also don't know where crack was first developed. It is one of the mysteries of the crack business that's yet to be unraveled. Crack has appeared in different forms in different places since the early 1980s, according to some reports from patients. For example, a form of crack, known as "rock" was seen on the West Coast in the early 1980s. Some teens say that they knew people who freebased and made crack up to three years ago. But in general, crack didn't find its way into those little vials and a ready market until recently.

So, how bad is crack from a crime standpoint? There are reports in the press of an increase in crime linked to crack and an increase in robberies in suburbia. To find the answer we asked Agent Stutman for his firsthand assessment: Is crack—and the crime it's causing—overplayed in the media?

"Absolutely not," he says emphatically. "If anything, it's worse. The key is that crack is a self-marketing product. Just think how Madison Avenue would like to have a bar of soap that *made* you buy it every time it was used up. That's what crack is like. You have to go back for more and more. Nothing could be worse from the stand-point of the growth of crack."

That's the true story of crack today. The only question left to ask is, How do we get crack out of our towns? We'll try to answer that crucial question in the next chapter.

·8·
Getting Crack Out of Your Town

The only way to get crack out of your town is to make your town totally drug-free. Crack is unique, but when it comes to stopping it, the solution is the same as for all drug use. Drug abuse can only be stopped by reducing the demand for drugs. Stopping drugs must begin with individuals, each of us.

Fortunately, an awareness that crack is so dangerous has moved many people to take a stand against drugs. As the crack epidemic has surfaced, communities have begun to mobilize. We've seen local block associations sponsor marches, schools put on anticrack days, states declare anticrack weeks, and mayors declare a "D Day in the War on Drugs." And, as everyone knows, the politicians have made the war on drugs their number-one priority. On October 26, 1986, President Reagan signed into law a $1.7 billion Omnibus Drug Enforcement Education and Control Act, which is designed to put some teeth back into the war on drugs. The bill increased penalties for drug traffickers and provided funding for more law-enforcement efforts and over $500 million for education in 1988 and 1989.

But laws aren't effective without genuine public support. The truth is that the war on drugs is first and foremost every person's responsibility. And that battle has to be fought at home first before it can be fought on the streets of your community.

WHAT TO DO FIRST

The first thing to do is learn everything you can about drugs and addiction. You may have used them yourself, or you may never have seen an illicit drug. Whatever you think you know about drugs from the media or from your own experience is probably out of date, perhaps incorrect, or just not enough. Information about addiction has changed over the years. Understanding the disease concept of addiction, the role of denial, and enabling are crucial to comprehending the addictive process.

Furthermore, your attitudes about drugs must be looked at and evaluated. They may be colored by your past experiences or your lack of knowledge. These attitudes, whether you know it or not, are often passed on to your family or friends. For example:

- Drugs are a necessary part of being a teenager.
- In order to learn how to be an adult, you need to learn how to use drugs successfully as a teenager.
- You need to drink or use drugs to be accepted socially by others.

In addition, we hear people whose lives haven't been touched by drug abuse who say things like, "It's part of the price we pay for living in a free country." But is it? Drug use is such a difficult problem that it's often easier to ignore or rationalize it than to cope with it. There is no reason to say that we have to trade our system of government to be free of drugs!

Comments like that show how little people understand the nature of drugs and their power to addict. As Dr. Mark Gold says, "Drugs addict people because drugs are addicting." Until people accept the truth about drugs and reject the myths, we'll never get drugs like crack out of town.

Getting an education about drugs begins with motivation to find out all you can. If you aren't motivated by what you've read here, you can always consider a few more statistics. Sixty percent of our children try illicit drugs by the time they graduate from high school. It's amazing, in the face of the amount of drugs available, that the other 40 percent don't. And the main reason so many kids try drugs and become disabled by them is really a lot simpler than you think: No one has ever told most of them why *not* to use drugs!

Most kids learn about drugs in the same place they learn about sex and rock and roll. From their friends. As a result, they become their own experts on the subject. Once again, myth and misinformation are responsible for many people using drugs because kids think they are safe.

The sad fact is this: Kids—and adults—will use illegal drugs until we give them real, clear, informed reasons to say no.

You can begin educating yourself by attending community or group sessions with experts from local treatment centers. If there are none, organize a program yourself. There is a list of organizations at the back of this book that you can contact to get accurate information if you have no community resource.

THINK ABOUT THIS

What are some of the things you must learn about drugs?

1. First, learn the difference between the drugs of the past decades and the drugs of today. For example, do you know what Ecstasy is? Or PCP? Or do you know the cumulative effects of the litany of drugs used by the teenagers in chapter three?

2. Do you know what the biggest-selling drug in your town is? Talk to the police or a treatment specialist and find out what the problem really is all about where you live. Use that information when trying to convince others that a good education program is needed.

3. Find out what your kids think they know. One mother living in a small community of four thousand people was shocked to find out that her fourth grader had been offered drugs. Her daughter not only knew where to get drugs but how much they cost and even what the color of the cap on the crack vial meant. "I thought it had to do with the potency of the drug," she said, "but it really had to do with the source—the distributor!"

4. Find out what your friends and neighbors and other parents think. People who start antidrug programs in their communities are shocked to discover the depth of feelings among their peers.

People who are just as worried as you are may simply be waiting for someone to begin the process.

5. Find out what the policy of the school system is in regard to drugs. Every school system in the USA should have a written policy about drug use. But very few have any sort of policy at all. And do you know why? Because many educators find it easier to tolerate kids on drugs who are not disruptive than to confront the damage done by drugs. Many parents are embarrassed to admit there is a problem in *their* kid's school by instituting a drug education or counseling program.

WHAT TO TELL KIDS ABOUT DRUGS

After you've educated yourself and learned as much as you can about drugs, then you have to take the next step. Stop drugs in your own home. This is going to be very difficult for many parents. Kids emulate adult behavior, and to them smoking, drinking, and taking drugs are all the same. After all, Mom and Dad have a few cocktails before dinner and they may smoke cigarettes. They may even have joked about their own drug use in the sixties.

Kids always argue, "Well, you do it, why can't I?"

Here's how you can reach kids who say that to you.

1. When you talk to anyone about drugs—including kids—be honest. Tell them the truth. Don't preach. There are too many anti-this and anti-that preachers out there talking about the evils of everything from rock lyrics to junk food. Drugs aren't the same. Drugs are much more serious and complicated. If you explain how drugs damage the body and how they can retard a developing central nervous system or reproductive system in an adolescent, they will listen.

Teenagers especially won't respond if you say, "If you take drugs you'll die." Potential fatal results of one's actions don't mean very much to young people. In fact, many are attracted to a drug like crack *just because* of its potential threat. They like the threat, the danger.

You have to plant a doubt in a kid's mind about what they think they know about drugs. They must see that you know more about the subject than their friends. Facts will give them a reason just to say no when confronted with the opportunity to use drugs. Then you have to take advantage of what Lee Dogoloff, Executive Director of the American Council for Drug Education, calls "teachable moments." If, for example, there's a news report on drugs—follow it up with a discussion—not a lecture. If something happens in your neighborhood or a community problem surfaces, take advantage of that moment to reinforce the information you've given them.

The war on the homefront is not a one-shot battle. Kids are going to have to make their own decisions. Parents of teenagers know that they can't make the decisions for them, so their best hope is that the kids will make a "knowing decision."

2. What about your own drug use? It's a question that anyone who hopes to get crack or any drug out of town has to deal with. There is no precise answer because all of us must cope with our own habits. But here are a few strategies to use.

Many parents have said, "Okay, we're going to have a family attack on cigarettes." In this instance, parents agree to give up smoking and kids must agree not to smoke or drink or do drugs.

Or, parents can decide that they will not smoke or drink in front of children. Many parents see this as the best compromise, and for many it's the only way to avoid confrontation over the subject.

Another answer is also possible. You may tell kids that smoking or drinking is not good, but point out that you are an adult and that these activities affect adults differently. Remind them that smoking, drinking, or taking drugs is an illegal activity for teenagers and is therefore unacceptable. You might mention that you wish you hadn't started smoking and urge them at least to postpone a decision to try any of these activities until they are eighteen or twenty-one. You may also point out to them how certain activities become addictive and that you have found it difficult to give up this addiction.

I often ask parents and loved ones to ask themselves the question, "How much do you value your teenager's life and well-being? Do you value it enough to give up drug and alcohol use while they are in their teenage years?" This is a small price to pay for what may have a big payoff for being a drug-free home.

3. Another thing to do is to make sure that your kids are not unwittingly put into situations where they can't escape. They may be going to a party where they don't expect to see drugs, but they appear anyway. You must make sure that parties are supervised. And that doesn't mean that the parents are in another wing of the house. Many communities have gotten parents together to pledge cooperation in keeping drugs and alcohol out of teen parties. In some communities parents sign pledges that they will not have any parties where drugs or alcohol are allowed, or if drugs are found the teen's parents are called.

IF THEY USE DRUGS

What should you do if you find out your kids have used drugs? This situation can provoke shock, guilt, anger, and even denial. In fact, that wall of denial is almost always the first reaction to the signs and symptoms that kids give off. These symptoms of drug use, described in chapter four, can't be ignored.

If you discover your kids are using drugs and you admit that it is happening to you, step back if you can. Don't overreact. Thomas Gleaton, executive director of PRIDE, says "I usually tell parents to take a deep breath, try to relax, and understand that this is something that can be taken care of." With education and a clear, sympathetic attitude, a parent can cope with a kid on drugs. Kids have to understand, says Gleaton, that you do care. "Tell them, 'I care too much about you to let you do this to yourself.'"

LET'S RECAP

If you can remember the following, you can help get drugs out of your town:

- Don't believe for a minute that drugs *aren't* in your town, your schools, or maybe in your own home. The damage to a community caused by drugs and the power of drugs like crack are far too great to ignore.

- To get crack out of your town or to stop your kids from killing themselves with alcohol and tobacco, you have to attack the wall of denial and indifference around you. Use education, facts, and reason as your weapons. Draw on community or regional resources as your allies. Don't miss an opportunity to reinforce the message. Help your kids, their peers, and your friends develop the ability to say no.
- Drugs will not go away on their own. Drug use is not a self-curing disease. Drugs like crack take over the entire body and possess it. The body becomes a vessel for the drug. The mind becomes a chemical messenger center for its ongoing damage. The saddest thing we ever heard from a teenager in treatment is this: "My drug use was so great that I don't remember much from the last two years of my life."

There's no reason except our own apathy, denial, or lack of education that any young person should be robbed of these vital teenage years.

• 9 •

Teach Your Kids to Say No to Crack

This entire book is about the effects of drugs like crack and what they can do to you and your family. It's also about what you can do to prevent drugs from coming into your town and your home. But the reality of the drug epidemic in America today is that you can't be everywhere to monitor your children. Ultimately, it's their choice. So how do you prepare them to say no to drugs?

There aren't any simple answers or ten easy rules to post on the refrigerator. But there are some specific guidelines you can create to equip your children to resist the peer pressure to use drugs. Not surprisingly, these have to be part of an overall approach to family life. To develop these guidelines and create a tailored approach that works for you, ask yourself a series of questions. How you answer them will help you help your kids learn to say no to drugs.

First look at yourself and what type of role model you present:

1. How do you use medication? Make your attitude clear to your children. If you don't take the pills a physician gives you absolutely correctly, then you are setting a bad example about the power and danger of medication or drugs of any kind. Always destroy the medicine you don't use and discard the bottle. Don't leave old medicines around the house.

2. Do you take a tranquilizer or grab a drink in front of your

children whenever the tensions of life rise? This is another bad example for children, who will interpret this as a sign that life's problems can be solved by artificial solutions. Avoid this behavior because children are very quick to pick up on it.

3. Do you have a "drug policy" at home? Just as we urge businesses to have a clear-cut policy on drugs, we also urge parents to have a mutually agreeable policy about the use of alcohol, cigarettes, and illegal drugs. Spend some time with the family discussing it whenever you can. You have to take a very strong stand against smoking, alcohol, and drugs and make it stick. But if it's to be a successful policy it has to be clarified for the parent as well as the child.

4. Do you know what to do if you find your child has used drugs? Fight and fight hard if you discover your child using drugs, cigarettes, or alcohol. If you think they are using drugs, search their rooms. If they are given alcohol at someone else's house, call the parents of that person and protest in the strongest possible terms. You must let your children know where you stand.

Remember, also, that you can't be successful without consistent stands on other rules. For example, if you set standards for schoolwork in order to allow them to be involved in extracurricular activities, don't modify that stance. The same goes for curfew and other rules around the house. If you have special family time—keep it. Don't go play golf or tennis or work if you can avoid it during these special family times.

5. Have you evaluated your children's peers? One theme of this book is the concept of denial. Be suspicious of any changes in behavior or groups of friends, and don't let up until you get an answer that satisfies you. A parent's responsibility is to be aware. If you think something is going on, ask questions. Be suspicious first and relieved second.

6. Have you missed any teachable moments? This applies to almost any activity with a child. For example, if you pass an accident on the highway, that's an opportunity to review safety on the road. The same applies to walking down the street and seeing someone smoking a joint. Use these moments to point out the negative impact that drugs can have. And remember that part of teaching includes emotional experiences. Help your child to

identify feelings and reactions to events. Remember that drugs affect feelings.

7. How have you educated your children about drugs? Have you given them enough factual information? How do you know if you have? Here's the test: If your kids know enough about drugs and their effects that they can walk away from a place where drugs are being used, then they have a good chance to say no each time drugs are offered. If they stay—even if they don't use the drug— they become desensitized to the dangers and this may lead to use later.

8. Have you helped them develop a good enough self-image to say no? Most kids, when exposed to drugs, have to make a tough choice: take the drug or lose a potential friend. Is your child strong enough to resist the challenge of his peers? Is he strong enough to lose those people? When teaching them about drugs and drug myths, keep these goals in mind.

9. Have you made clear to them the "other" consequences of using drugs? Do they understand the damage it will do to their family and family life? Kids who can say no to drugs are those for whom loss of the family is far more important than loss of a group of friends. If you've educated children about drugs, been a good role model, and equipped them with enough facts, they will, more often than not, say no to drugs.

10. Have you remained open to learning from your children? In today's rapidly changing world, our child's experiences at a given age are dramatically different from ours. Children need guidance but it must be from a standpoint of understanding. Listen to your child and talk to him about what life is like for him. We can learn how to guide someone better if we know what and who we are really guiding.

In the end, getting your kids to learn how to say no to drugs isn't something that you do around the dining room table on a rainy Saturday afternoon. It is a process that starts as early as you think your kids can understand the information—kindergarten is a good place to begin for most kids.

So begin today!

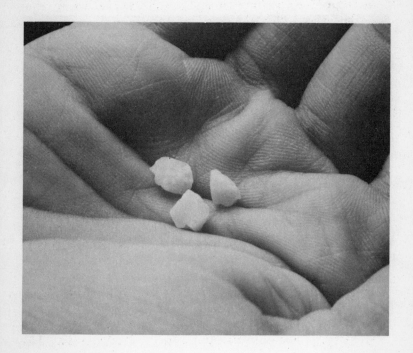

Crack rocks: Less than a handful of these tiny crack rocks can start someone in the addictive process. These three pieces of crack together affect the user less than thirty minutes and cost five to ten dollars each.

(Courtesy of Fair Oaks Hospital at Boca/Delray, Florida.)

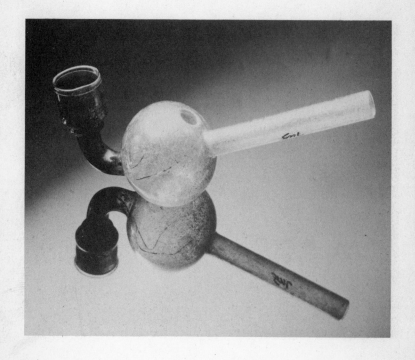

Crack pipe: A typical pipe used to smoke crack. The rocks are placed in the bowl and the smoke is drawn through the water in the large chamber. The smoke enters the lungs and moves rapidly—in about three to five seconds—to the brain. These pipes cost about $10.

(Courtesy Fair Oaks Hospital at Boca/Delray, Florida.)

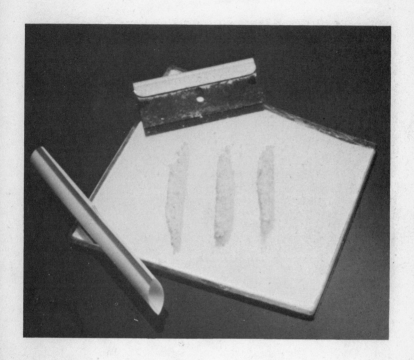

Cocaine powder: Three "lines" of cocaine, chopped into a fine powder with the blade, are laid out on a smooth, hard surface, ready to be sniffed through the straw. Cocaine powder is absorbed intranasally and begins its effect within a few minutes. Cocaine powder is also sniffed with special "coke spoons" and through rolled up bills.
(Courtesy Fair Oaks Hospital at Boca/Delray, Florida.)

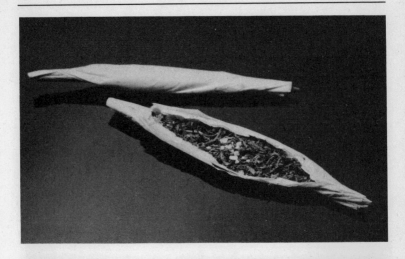

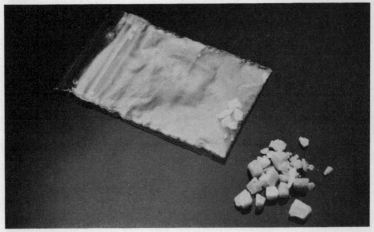

Two "joints" or marijuana cigarettes laced with fragments of crack.
(Courtesy Fair Oaks Hospital at Boca/Delray, Florida.)
Crack bag: Crack dealers rarely carry more than this amount—
about $75.00 worth of crack—to avoid prosecution for "trafficking."
This amount here is broken out into small vials, foil pouches, or tiny
jars for sale on the street.
(Courtesy Fair Oaks Hospital at Boca/Delray, Florida.)

Referrals[1]

TOLL-FREE INFORMATION

1-800-554-KIDS—THE NATIONAL FEDERATION OF PARENTS FOR DRUG-FREE YOUTH (NFP).

1-800-241-9746—PRIDE DRUG INFORMATION LINE.

1-800-638-2045—NATIONAL INSTITUTE ON DRUG ABUSE (NIDA), U.S. DEPARTMENT OF HEALTH AND HUMAN SERVICES.

1-800-662-HELP—NIDA HOTLINE.

1-800-COCAINE—COCAINE HELPLINE.

GENERAL READINGS AND VIDEOTAPES

The publications in the following list that are followed by an (a) or (b) are available from these organizations:

(a) National Federation of Parents for Drug-Free Youth (NFP), 8730 Georgia Avenue, Suite 200, Silver Spring, MD 20910. Telephone toll-free nationwide 1-800-554-KIDS, or in the Washington, D.C., area, 585-KIDS.

(b) Parents' Resource Institute for Drug Education, Inc. (PRIDE), Woodruff Bldg., Suite 1002, 100 Edgewood Avenue, Atlanta, GA 30303. Telephone toll-free nationwide 1-800-241-9746.

1. From *What Works: Schools Without Drugs*, United States Department of Education, 1986.

Bachman, Jerald G., Lloyd D. Johnson, and Patrick M. O'Malley. *Drug Use Among American High School Students, College Students, and Other Young Adults: National Trends Through 1985*. The National Institute on Drug Abuse, 1986. Rockville, MD 20857, ADM 86-1450. Single copies are available free.

Courtwatch Manual. Washington Legal Foundation, 1705 N Street, NW, Washington, D.C. 20036. Enclose $2.00 for postage and handling.

Dupont, Robert, Jr. *Getting Tough on Gateway Drugs*. American Psychiatric Press Inc., 1984. (a) (b)

Gold, Mark S. *800-COCAINE*. New York: Bantam Books, 1984.

How to Talk to Your Kids About Growing Up Without Drugs and Alcohol. Videotape. (a)

MacDonald, Donald I. *Adolescent Drug and Alcohol Abuse*. Year Book Publishers, 1984. 35 East Wacker Drive, Chicago, IL 60601. Telephone 1-800-621-9262.

Manatt, Marsha. *Parents, Peers and Pot II: Parents in Action*. U.S. Department of Health and Human Services, 1983. $1.00 (b)

Newton, Miller. *Gone Way Down, Teenage Drug-Use Is a Disease*. American Studies Press, 1981. (a)

Polich, J. Michael, et al. *Strategies for Controlling Adolescent Drug Use*. The Rand Corporation, 1984. 1700 Main Street, P.O. Box 2138, Santa Monica, CA 90406-2138.

Polson, Beth, and Miller Newton. *Not My Kid*. Avon Books, 1984. (b)

Scott, Sharon. *Peer Pressure Reversal*. Human Resource Development Center, 1985. Amherst, MA. (a) (b)

Team Up for Drug Prevention With America's Young Athletes. Drug Enforcement Administration, Public Affairs Staff, 1405 Eye Street, NW, Washington, D.C. 20537. Free.

Tobias, Joyce. *Kids and Drugs: A Handbook for Parents and Professionals*. Panda Press, 1986. 4111 Watkins Trail, Annandale, VA 22003. Telephone (703) 750-9285.

FREE CATALOGS OF DRUG ABUSE PUBLICATIONS

Comp Care Publications. A source for pamphlets, books, and charts on drug and alcohol abuse, chemical awareness, and self-help. Telephone 1-800-328-3330.

Hazelden Educational Materials. A source for pamphlets and books on drug abuse and alcoholism and curriculum materials for drug prevention. Telephone 1-800-328-9000.

SCHOOL AND COMMUNITY RESOURCES

Alcohol and Drug Abuse Education Program, U.S. Department of Education. For information, write to the U.S. Department of Education,

Alcohol and Drug Abuse Education Program, 400 Maryland Avenue, SW, Washington, D.C. 20202-4101.

American Council on Drug Education (ACDE), 5820 Hubbard Drive, Rockville, MD 20852. Telephone (301) 984-5700.

Committees of Correspondence, Inc. Membership is $15.00. 57 Conant Street, Room 113, Danvers, MA 09123. Telephone (617) 774-2641.

Fair Oaks Hospital, 19 Prospect Street, Summit, NJ 07901. Telephone 1-800-COCAINE.

Families in Action. $10.00 for 4 issues. 3845 North Druid Hills Road, Suite 300, Decatur, GA 30033. Telephone (404) 325-5799.

Narcotics Education, Inc. 6830 Laurel Street, NW, Washington, D.C. 20012. Telephone 1-800-548-8700, or in the Washington, D.C., area, call (202) 722-6740.

National Federation of Parents for Drug-Free Youth (NFP). 8730 Georgia Avenue, Suite 200, Silver Spring, MD 20910. Telephone: Washington, D.C., area (301) 585-KIDS, or toll-free hotline 1-800-554-KIDS.

National Institute on Alcoholism and Alcohol Abuse (NIAAA), P.O. Box 2345, Rockville, MD 20852. Telephone (301) 468-2600.

National Institute on Drug Abuse (NIDA), Room 10-A-43, 5600 Fishers Lane, Rockville, MD 20852. Telephone (301) 443-6500.

Parents' Resource Institute for Drug Education, Inc. (PRIDE). Woodruff Bldg., Suite 1002, 100 Edgewood Avenue, Atlanta, GA 30303. Telephone 1-800-241-9746.

Phoenix House. 164 W. 74th Street, New York, NY 10023. Telephone (212) 595-5810.

Target. National Federation of State High School Associations, 11724 Plaza Circle, P.O. Box 20626, Kansas City, MO 64195. Telephone (816) 464-5400.

Toughlove. P.O. Box 1069, Doylestown, PA 18901. Telephone (215) 348-7090.

ADOLESCENT DRUG REHABILITATION PROGRAMS

To find programs, call your city or county substance abuse or mental health agency, hospitals, schools, local hotlines listed in the Yellow Pages, and the hotlines listed previously. It is best to visit prospective programs and to talk with people who have completed the program.

Sources

"America on Drugs." *U.S. News & World Report,* July 28, 1986.

Anker, Antoinette L., and T. J. Crowley. "Use of Contingency Contracts in Specialty Clinics for Cocaine Abuse," NIDA Research Monograph Series, Problems of Drug Dependence, 1981.

Annitto, William J., and M. S. Gold. "The Fair Oaks Hospital Cocaine Treatment Program," *Journal of Substance Abuse and Treatment,* vol. 1: 223–26, 1984.

"Battling the Enemy Within." *Time,* Mar. 17, 1986.

Belkin, Lisa. "Choosing Antidrug Therapy for Teenagers," *The New York Times,* Sept. 15, 1984.

Bensinger, Peter B. "Drugs in the Workplace: A Commentary," *Behavioral Sciences & the Law,* vol. 3, no. 4: 441–53, 1985.

Bloch, Jeff. "So What? Everybody's Doing It," *Forbes,* Aug. 11, 1986.

Brinkley, Joel. "Drug Crops Are Up in Export Nations State Dept. Says," *The New York Times,* Feb. 15, 1985.

———. "Drug Production in U.S. Is Reported at Record Levels," *The New York Times,* June 2, 1986.

———. "House Panel Finds Failure in World Drug Control," *The New York Times,* June 19, 1984.

Byars, Tom. "Educate to Eradicate," *Security Management,* December 1983.

Chilnick, Lawrence D., ed. *The Coke Book.* New York: Berkley Books, 1984.

———. *The Little Black Pill Book.* New York: Bantam Books, 1983.

Cohen, S. "Cocaine: Acute Medical and Psychiatric Complications," *Psychiatric Annals* 14(10): 728–32, 1984.

"Crack." *Time,* June 2, 1986.

"Crack & Crime." *Newsweek,* June 16, 1986.

"Crashing on Cocaine." *Time,* Apr. 11, 1983.

Dackis, C. A., and M. S. Gold. "Bromocriptine as Treatment of Cocaine Abuse," *The Lancet,* 1151–52, May 18, 1985.

———. "New Concepts in Cocaine Addiction: The Dopamine Depletion Hypothesis," *Neuroscience & Behavioral Reviews,* vol. 9: 496–77, 1985.

"'Doing' Cocaine: A Victim's Road to Ruin." *U.S. News & World Report,* May 16, 1983.

"Drinking on the Job." *The Wall Street Journal,* May 7, 1985.

"Drug Abuse in Sports: Denial Fuels the Problem." *The Physician and Sportsmedicine,* April 1982.

"Drugs: A Plan to Curb Demand." *Newsweek,* July 28, 1986.

"Easing Cocaine Withdrawal." *Medical World News,* Nov. 11, 1985.

Ercolano, Doreen, et al. "Crack Use: Creeping Towards Long Island," *Suffolk Life,* Aug. 6, 1986.

"The Evil Empire." *Newsweek,* Feb. 25, 1985.

Franklin, Ben A. "Mayors Plan Day to Focus on Drugs," *The New York Times,* Sept. 9, 1986.

Gay, George R. "You've Come a Long Way Baby! Coke Time for the New American Lady of the Eighties," *Journal of Psychoactive Drugs,* vol. 13, no. 4, Oct.–Dec. 1981.

Gold, Mark S. "Cocaine Is Clearly Addictive," *Alcoholism & Addiction,* Jan.–Feb. 1986.

———. "Dangers in Young People Smoking Pot," *Physician & Patient,* January 1983.

———. "Don't Snort It—Sneeze on It," *USA Today,* Nov. 28, 1984.

———. *800-COCAINE.* New York: Bantam Books, 1984.

———. *The Facts about Drugs and Alcohol.* New York: Bantam Books, 1986.

———. "Pot Is Gateway Drug for Adolescents," *Alcoholism & Addiction,* Mar.–Apr. 1986.

———. "Wealthy Cocaine Users," *Alcoholism & Addiction,* July–Aug. 1985.

Gold, Mark S., and W. S. Rea. "The Role of Endorphins in Opiate Addiction, Opiate Withdrawal and Recovery," *Psychiatric Clinics of North America,* vol. 6, September 1983.

Gold, Mark S., and K. Vereby. "Psychopharmacology of Cocaine," *Psychiatric Annals on Cocaine.* N. J.: Slack, 1984.

———. "The Psychopharmacology of Cocaine," *Psychiatric Annals* 14(10): 714–23.

Gold, Mark S., L. Semlitz, C. A. Dackis and I. Extein. "The Adolescent Cocaine Epidemic," *Seminars in Adolescent Medicine,* 1(4): 303–09, 1985.

Gold, Mark S., A. M. Washton, C. A. Dackis and J. C. Chatlos. "New

Treatments for Opiate and Cocaine Users: But What About Marijuana?" *Psychiatric Annals* 16(4): 221–24, 1986.

Grafton, Samuel, ed. "Substance Abuse Report," vol. XVI, no. 3: March 1985.

Helfrich, Antoinette A., Thomas J. Crowley, Carol A. Atkinson and Robin D. L. Post. "A Clinical Profile of 136 Cocaine Abusers," National Institute of Drug Abuse, *Problems of Drug Dependence*, 1983.

Hodgoson, Harriet W. *A Parent's Survival Guide*. Center City, MN: Hazelden Foundation, 1986.

Hoover, Paul E., Nestor B. Kowalsky and Richard L. Masters. "An Employee Assistance Program for Professional Pilots (An Eight Year Review)." Denver, CO: Airline Pilots Association, 1982.

Hoover, R. David, ed. *Drugs of Abuse*. Washington, D.C.: U.S. Govt. Printing Office, 1985.

"How Drugs Sap the Nation's Strength." *U.S. News & World Report*, May 16, 1983.

James, Stacy V. "Detecting Drugs in the Body," *The New York Times*, Mar. 22, 1986.

Jonas, J. M., and M. S. Gold. "Cocaine Abuse and Eating Disorders," *Lancet* 1 (8477): 390, 1986.

Khantzian, E. J., and N. J. Khantzian. "Cocaine Addiction: Is There a Psychological Predisposition?" *Psychiatric Annals* 14(10): 753–59, 1984.

"Kids and Cocaine." *Newsweek*, Mar. 17, 1986.

Kline, David. "The Anatomy of Addiction," *Equinox*, Sept.–Oct. 1985.

Kroll, Larry J. "The Cocaine Epidemic," *EAP Digest*, Nov.–Dec. 1985.

Lawn, John C. "Drugs in America." San Francisco, CA: Commonwealth Club speech, Feb. 13, 1986.

Lombardi, John. "Cocaine: Chic, Fun . . . Deadly," *Daily News*, Jan. 25, 1984.

———. "The Great White Hoax," *Sunday News Magazine*, Jan. 22, 1984.

Lubasch, Arnold H. "Ex-U.S. Lawyer Admits Stealing Drugs and Cash," *The New York Times*, Oct. 19, 1985.

McClellan, Thomas A., et al. "Is Treatment for Substance Abuse Effective?" *Journal of the American Medical Association*, vol. 247, no. 10: 1423–28, Mar. 12, 1982.

Macdonald, D. I., and D. Czechowicz. "Marijuana: A Pediatric Overview," *Psychiatric Annals*, 16(4): 215–18, 1986.

Malcolm, Andrew H. "Worried Citizens Are Joining Officials Around U.S. to Fight Spread of Crack," *The New York Times*, Sept. 14, 1986.

Maranto, Gina. "Coke: The Random Killer," *Discover*, March 1985.

Meddis, Sam, and Karen DeWitt. "Drug Force Targets Florida," *USA Today*, Oct. 1, 1984.

Meyers, Jim. "Finding the Right Help for a Teen Addict," *USA Today*, Sept. 17, 1986.

Milgram, Gail G. *What, When & How to Talk to Children about Alcohol and Other Drugs,* Center City, MN: Hazelden Foundation.

Minzesheimer, Bob, and Sam Meddis. "Baby Boomers Switch from Pot to Coke," *USA Today,* Nov. 28, 1984.

Mule, S. J. "The Pharmacodynamics of Cocaine Abuse," *Psychiatric Annals* 14(10): 747–49, 1984.

"Multiple Drug Abuse Escalates." *Medical World News,* July 22, 1985.

Newton, Miller. "Adolescent Drug Use as a Disease," in *Gone Way Down.* American Studies Press, 1981.

O'Boyle, Thomas F. "More Firms Require Drug Tests," *The Wall Street Journal,* Aug. 8, 1985.

Ostrow, Robert J. "Worker Theft Widespread—Survey," *Los Angeles Times,* June 11, 1983.

Perry, David. "The Pharmacology of Addiction and Drug Dependence," *PharmChem Newsletter,* July 1976.

Pope, Harrison G., et al. "Drug Use and Lifestyle among College Undergraduates," *Archive of General Psychiatry,* vol. 38: 588–91, May 1981.

"Reach." Montreal: Royal Bank of Canada.

Reilly, Patrick. "Cocaine Plagues Corporate Centers," *Crain's New York Business,* Feb. 25, 1985.

Ricks, Thomas E. "The Cocaine Business: Big Risks and Profits, High Labor Turnover," *The Wall Street Journal,* June 30, 1986.

———. "Eastern Airlines Baggage Handlers in Miami Indicted in Cocaine Importation Case," *The Wall Street Journal,* Sept. 29, 1986.

Satchell, Michael. "Does Hollywood Sell Drugs to Kids?" *Parade,* July 21, 1985.

Schmeck, Harold M. "Drug Abuse in America: Widening Array Brings New Perils," *The New York Times,* Mar. 22, 1983.

Schmidt, William E. "Police Say Use of Crack Is Moving to Small Towns and Rural Areas," *The New York Times,* Sept. 10, 1986.

Schnoll, S. H., and A. N. Daghestani. "Treatment of Marijuana Abuse," *Psychiatric Annals,* 16(4): 249–54, 1986.

Schroeder, Donald D. "Snow Fever," *The Plain Truth,* January 1985.

Schuckit, Marc A. *Drug and Alcohol Abuse,* 2d ed. New York: Plenum Press, 1984.

Schwartz, Rich H. "Marijuana: A Crude Drug with a Spectrum of Underappreciated Toxicity," *Pediatrics,* vol. 73, no. 4: 455–58, April 1985.

Schwartz, Rich H., P. R. Cohen and G. Blair. "Identifying and Coping with Drug-Using Adolescents: Some Guidelines for Pediatricians and Parents," *Pediatrics in Review,* vol. 5, no. 5: 133–139, November 1985.

Schwartz, Rich H., and Richard L. Hawks. "Laboratory Detection of Marijuana Use," *Journal of the American Medical Association,* vol. 254, no. 6: 788–92, August 1985.

Semlitz, L., and M. S. Gold. "Adolescent Drug Abuse: Diagnosis, Treatment and Prevention," *Psychiatric Clinics of North America,* 1986.

"Senate Approves Bill to Combat Drugs." *The New York Times*, Oct. 1, 1986.

Shafer, Jack. "The War on Drugs Is Over. The Government Has Lost," *Inquiry*, February 1984.

Shenon, Phillip. "24 Task Forces to Fight Crack Sought by Meese," *The New York Times*, Oct. 3, 1986.

Shriver, Jerry. "Employers Are Helping Addicted Workers," *USA Today*, Jan. 12, 1984.

Siegel, R. K. "Cocaine Smoking Disorders: Diagnosis and Treatment," *Psychiatric Annals*, 14(10): 753–59, 1984.

Smilon, Marvin, and Dick Rosenberg. "Four Wall Street Brokers Held in Coke Ring," *New York Post*, May 7, 1986.

Smith, D. E. "Cocaine Abuse." New York: Paper Presented at the Women & Work Conference, November 1982.

Smith, D. E., and D. R. Wesson. "Cocaine," *Journal of Psychedelic Drugs*, vol. 10, no. 4: Oct.–Dec. 1978.

———. "Consideration of Cocaine Dosage," *Journal of Psychedelic Drugs*, vol. 10, no. 4: Oct–Dec. 1978.

Smith, David E., ed., et al. "Substance Abuse in the Workplace." San Francisco, CA: Haight-Ashbury Publications, 1984.

Span, Paula. "Treating the Affluent Drug Addict," *USA Today*, Jan. 9, 1984.

Sperling, Dan. "New Drug Big Risk to Young," *USA Today*, Dec. 10, 1985.

"The Surgeon General's Warning on Marijuana." *Morbidity and Mortality Report*, vol. 31, no. 31: Aug. 13, 1982.

"Team MDs Call for Mandatory Drug Tests." *American Medical News*, Mar. 14, 1986.

Thornton, Mary. "Heroin and Cocaine Use Rising, Panel Reports," *The Washington Post*, Mar. 5, 1986.

Trice, Harrison M., and Janice M. Beyer. "A Study of Union-Management Cooperation in a Long-Standing Alcoholism Program," *Contemporary Drug Problems*, Summer, 1982.

"Trouble in the Valley." *Newsweek*, Feb. 25, 1985.

"Trying to Say 'No.'" *Newsweek*, Aug. 11, 1986.

"U.S. Campaign to Fight Drugs in State Backed." *The New York Times*, June 15, 1984.

Washton, Arnold M. "Structured Outpatient Treatment of Cocaine Abuse," *Advances in Alcohol and Substance Abuse*, 1985.

———. "Recent Trends in Cocaine Abuse: A View from the National Hotline," *Advances in Alcohol and Substance Abuse*, 1985.

Webb, Dan K. "Recent Developments in White Collar Crime," *Vital Speeches of the Day*, vol. 51, no. 6:175–78, Jan. 1, 1985.

Werner, Leslie M. "Crime Panel Told of Cocaine Abuse," *The New York Times*, Nov. 28, 1984.

Wilbur, Robert. "Kicking Cocaine," *Chicago Tribune*, Feb. 23, 1986.

Wilford, B. B. *Drug Abuse: A Guide for the Primary Care Physician*. Chicago: American Medical Association, 1981.

Wilkinson, Peter. "Cocaine: USA's Problem Line," *Women's Wear Daily*, Jan. 8, 1986.

"The Young Drinkers: Teenagers and Alcohol." Hollywood, FL: Health Communications, Inc., 1978.

DATE DUE